ETHICS

THE PATIENT'S CHARTER

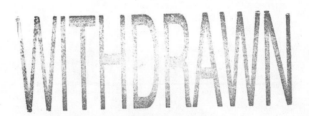

Also in this series

ETHICS

THE PATIENT'S CHARTER

Edited by

Verena Tschudin BSc(Hons), RGN, RM,
Dip Counselling

Illustrations by Richard Smith

Scutari Press • London

First published 1995

British Library Cataloguing in Publication Data

Tschudin, Verena
    Patient's Charter. – (Ethics Series)
    I. Title II. Series
    174.2

    ISBN   1–873853–30–0

Phototypeset by Intype, London

Printed and bound by Athenæum Press Ltd.,
Gateshead, Tyne & Wear.

Contents

Contributors

Peter Baddeley MRCP, MRCGP, DRCOG, DGM

Independent General Practitioner, Stroud, Gloucestershire

Angeline Burke

Development Officer, Association of Community Health Councils for England and Wales

Adrian Childs MSc, RMN, RGN, DipN(Lond)

Quality Assurance Nurse, Maudsley Hospital, London

Nigel Ellis

Research/Information Officer, Association of Community Health Councils for England and Wales

Ben Griffith

Information Officer (Health Policy), Association of Community Health Councils for England and Wales

Verena Tschudin BSc(Hons), RGN, RM,
Dip Counselling

Senior Lecturer, University of East London

Andrew Wall BA(Hons), MSc, FHSM

Senior Fellow, Health Services Management Centre, University of Birmingham

Preface

The last volume in this series is unusual, in that it deals with just one subject.

The Patient's Charter is one of those topics that elicit a response when mentioned: people either like it or they do not, but they are rarely indifferent to it. This is so whether they are patients and clients or purchasers and providers. The whole concept of charters is new, and any newly imposed ideas often elicit, first of all, a hostile response, especially when it means having to change one's ways of thinking and acting. For those who like new ideas, the Charter may come as a liberation and an authorisation to change outmoded ways.

In terms of ethics, the Patient's Charter is specifically about the rights of patients and clients. Implicit in the Charter is, therefore, that those who provide the rights have and take responsibilities, so that the rights can and will exist. For nursing, this means specifically the named nurse (Charter standard no. 8). But while most of the other rights apply more specifically to doctors and managers, nurses have responsibilities to see that patients do not miss out on any right.

A charter informs and shapes society in subtle and blunt ways. It is essentially in our behaviour to each other that ethical thinking and behaving is evident. Even when we consider that something is 'none of our business' it *is* our business because we are part of society. Sooner or later, we are all either at the receiving end or the giving end of care and thus experience a right as a responsibility or a responsibility as a right. The Patient's Charter is here whether we like it or not. We may, therefore, do well to see it not as a hostile intrusion, but as something useful and helpful for the whole of society.

Of all the volumes in this series, this one has been the most difficult to put together. The result is a collection of individual views and approaches to the Charter that are unlikely to be met together between book covers elsewhere. The authors have brought together their areas of interest, which differ widely, but all of them are concerned not to lose sight of the *raison d'être* of the Charter: the individual patient. As such, this book should be a useful contribution to the debate about charters in general and the NHS Patient's Charter in particular.

Verena Tschudin

CHAPTER 1

A Nurse's View

Adrian Childs

The first chapter in this volume looks at the Patient's Charter from one nurse's point of view. The author demonstrates an intimate knowledge of the Charter and an enthusiasm for its use that are far reaching.

The concept of the 'named nurse' has given nurses much food for thought, and this chapter addresses the issue with clarity. However, quality is also considered, as is the standpoint of the individual nurse who is not 'named'. These aspects are dealt with in a wide framework of nursing care, philosophy, education, ethics and the need for change and re-evaluation at all these levels.

This chapter attempts to examine the Patient's Charter (DoH, 1991) from a nurse's perspective. It does not seek to demonstrate how to implement such a Charter, but rather to explore the unwritten implications that the Patient's Charter has on nursing practice. Many of the concepts discussed here are not new: they have been considered in nursing literature for some time. However, the Charter necessitates that nurses cease to discuss the concepts and begin to incorporate them into their everyday practice.

The Patient's Charter is one of the central parts of the government's Citizen's Charter initiative. The Patient's Charter is perhaps the key concept in the government's programme to improve and modernise the delivery of health-care services to the public, while continuing to reaffirm the principles of the NHS. The document itself can be seen as politically motivated: it aims to move the NHS towards a market economy in line with the rest of the public sector and, as such, must be viewed in conjunction with other government initiatives, for example Caring for People and Working for Patients.

However, perhaps more importantly, the Patient's Charter provides both health-care workers and users of the health-care services with a formal quality monitoring tool. This is synonymous with ensuring that the public sector is more accountable for the service it provides and that monitoring the quality of that service is the concern of not only the provider, but also the user. This tool clearly identifies outcome measures to which health-care providers must aspire, in terms of the service that is provided and what users of that service can expect to receive.

The fact that the remit of this document is so wide, in terms of political implications, does not mean that nurses can or should leave its implementation, monitoring and further development to others; the opposite is, in fact, true. Nurses must be involved with this critical development in the NHS and health-care delivery. Nurses should work towards applying this Charter at three levels of functioning: as a group of professionals, as a group of nurses within an organisation and within their everyday, individual practice. To achieve success, nurses also need to be active at all levels: passivity will not implement the Charter effectively. Here is an opportunity to strengthen the nurses' position and for nurses actively to participate in the development of service delivery to the patient.

Nurses are, however, not able to perform such tasks alone. Health-care delivery is complex and is developing a more multidisciplinary focus, and, as such, to work in isolation would be detrimental to the Charter. A collaborative approach should be taken, working with other disciplines and service users.

The Patient's Charter is aimed at the general population, but many health-care services are specialist. It is, therefore, inappropriate to expect the Charter to be applied verbatim.

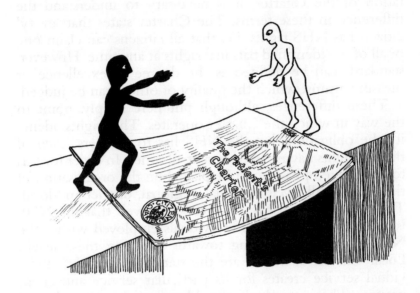

Different services care for different client groups, all of whom have different needs. It is essential that the implementation of the Charter accommodates these. According to service and client need, different aspects of the Charter will be emphasised in the various service areas.

It is perhaps, therefore, more appropriate to consider the underlying spirit of the Charter rather than focus on the specific rights and standards identified within it. This is not to say that nurses should not work towards achieving these but rather that they should aim to develop their practice to encompass the forward movement of health-care delivery, ensuring that it is patient focused and clearly measurable from both a user's and a provider's perspective.

The Patient's Charter is divided into two broad areas — rights and standards — at both a national and a local level.

In order that nurses can work towards effective implementation of the Charter, it is necessary to understand the difference in these terms. The Charter states that 'every' citizen has NHS rights, i.e. that all citizens can claim one or all of the identified national rights at any time. However, standards can be defined as the degree of excellence or measure against which the quality of others can be judged.

These differences, although put here simply, point to the way in which the Charter operates. The 'rights' identify the obligation that the NHS has to its users, each of the ten rights having to be met at all times. In order for this to happen, emphasis must be placed on the organisation of the NHS at all levels: national, regional, district and local. The national standards, however, are levels that the NHS is aiming to achieve. All individuals employed within the NHS should be working towards attaining these levels. Local Charter standards are the standards that each individual service creates for its particular service and client groups. These standards should reflect local needs and should again be considered as those which the service is aiming to achieve.

This chapter will consider how the Patient's Charter affects nursing practice and how nurses can work towards its successful implementation. However, rather than consider each right and standard in isolation, it aims to focus on the spirit of the Charter. It will identify three themes that are considered to be of importance in terms of nursing practice and the nursing profession: quality, the named nurse concept and the individual nurse practitioner. The overall aim of the discussion is to provide the reader with an attempt to look beyond the written word of the Charter and consider the implications that such a document has on a profession and its members in terms of practice and ethical considerations. Many nurses think of responsibility, advocacy, change, etc. as managerial problems and issues. However, they are essentially ethical aspects of professional work. This chapter highlights their interrelationships. By taking this approach, it is obvious that not all aspects of the Charter will be covered. However, it is hoped that the discussion will stimulate thought and encourage a wider and more analytical view in the implementation of such documents.

Quality

The Patient's Charter provides both health-care workers and users of health-care services with a formal quality monitoring tool. In order to examine this further, it is necessary to explore the concept of quality in relation to nursing.

The concern for quality has rapidly spread through the NHS. With the introduction of the government's white paper *Working for Patients* (DoH, 1989) the NHS has moved further towards a market economy and placed heavy emphasis on a consumer-oriented health-care service. It has further developed this concept with the introduction of the purchaser–provider scenario, and thus an element of competition has developed between providers (Avis, 1992). Quality has, therefore, become a major issue. Services are going to be compared not only in terms of price, but also in terms of the quality that is offered.

With what, then, does quality concern itself? The word 'quality' has been used in two very different ways. It has been used to describe levels of excellence; for example, one commonly hears about 'the quality press'. Alternatively, quality has been used to refer to the character of something, and in this way it is possible to describe the level of quality, i.e. good or bad.

Wilson-Barnett (1981) states that quality concerns itself with the value or benefit that can be derived from care. Quality is the degree of success which is achieved in reaching goals; it assumes evaluation of care. This definition focuses on the outcome or product of care. Care and caring are complex phenomena, and in nursing, they are often seen as the skills, the knowledge and the performance of tasks in an uncomplaining fashion. Tschudin (1992) purports that caring is more than this. The carer is in a relationship with the care-receiver, and this constitutes care and caring. Tschudin continues that those who receive care believe that what matters is how human the individuals providing the care are, rather than their expertise in performing tasks or their perceived knowledge. Barber (1991) explores caring through an experience of hospitalisation and stresses the importance of the therapeutic relationship in the concept of caring, supporting Tschudin's (1992) ideas.

Wilson-Barnett's (1981) definition, therefore, may be acceptable when looking specifically at tasks, knowledge base, efficiency and the results or products of care. All these things can be measured and, as such, can satisfy the nurse's role within the Patient's Charter. Statistics can be produced in relation to the Charter's rights and standards. However, if nurses consider much of their role to be caring, such a definition will not adequately meet their needs. As well as all the tangible things that nurses do, a definition of quality for nurses needs to consider the intangible: how to measure the level of success of the relationship between the nurse as carer and the patient as care-receiver. These intangible aspects include the elements that are vital to the therapeutic relationship, such as the ability to value the human condition, recognising the patient's individuality, the nurses' ability to incorporate patients as a resource and actively to encourage them to participate in their care, to work with them rather than do to them and to develop and honour openness, honesty and trust within the relationship, thus enabling the patient to feel valued. Taylor (1992) believes that the effects of describing nurses as dispensers of help and care only lead them to be stripped of the qualities that make them people and human. It is the essential nature of nurses as people that enhances the therapeutic relationship, which begins to offer meaning to the patient's health status and which must be considered when exploring quality.

Ellis (1988) takes a wider viewpoint and suggests that quality is the totality of features or characteristics of a product or service that bear on its ability to satisfy a given need, suggesting that quality is that which gives complete customer satisfaction. Such a definition considers both the process of the service and its outcome. However, confusion arises when attempts are made explicitly to identify the customer. Patients receive direct care, i.e. the services provided by nurses, and could, therefore, be considered, as the recipients of a service, as customers. However, the purchaser provides the finance necessary to offer the services and could, therefore, also be reasonably considered as the customer, as the services nurses provide are identified in contractual agreements.

The point of this discussion is to demonstrate that quality has different meanings to different groups of people. What quality means to a general manager may not represent the views of a group of clinicians. Perhaps, therefore, it is more appropriate not to offer a hard and fast definition but to accept that any services provided need to be monitored and evaluated; the generation of a meaning for quality needs to come from within that particular service. Such a definition must reflect the nurses' views and opinions and be an inherent part of their philosophy and functioning, while still incorporating the overall views of the organisation.

A definition that has proved useful and adaptable in the past is to consider quality as a nebulous concept, meaning no more and no less than a description of the nature and characteristics of a product or service. Although simplistic, such an explanation gives nurses the ability to use the concept of quality and adapt and relate it to the services they provide. This definition does not focus purely on the processes or outcomes of a service but enables nurses to encompass both issues. It is thus able to provide meaning to both nurses and patients alike. This is particularly relevant in relation to the Patient's Charter when we consider it to be a monitoring tool for both providers of services and patients.

The difficulty in establishing a universal definition of quality highlights the problems associated with monitoring the quality of services. The array of available definitions only demonstrates the numerous ways in which to implement, monitor and evaluate quality strategies. The Patient's Charter has identified one way forward, in setting nine national standards. One of the problems associated with quality assurance programmes is establishing clear, appropriate and acceptable standards. In health care, standards involve considering both the delivery and outcomes of care (Ellis and Whittington, 1993). To some extent, the Patient's Charter has achieved this. The standards are jargon-free and clearly understandable, measurable by both health-care professionals and patients alike. For example, national standard no. 6 states that for an outpatient appointment, 'you will be given a specific time and be seen within thirty minutes of that time'. This clearly states what the objective is and enables both the patient and health-care professional to establish whether or not it is achieved.

However, what the Charter does not do is examine process within its standards. Process standards explore the procedure for achieving an identified outcome. Nursing is, perhaps, the most developed health-care profession in considering process standards (Ellis and Whittington, 1993). This is essential in order to ensure that patients have a better understanding of the process of health care and are able to relate this information to their own individual experiences. For the benefit of both nursing and the patient, it is essential that we continue to develop process standards, particularly in relation to local Charter standards. This is even more important when considering the earlier discussion about defining quality. If, to nurses, the therapeutic relationship is integral to the delivery of nursing care, far more explicit process standards need to be developed, which focus on interpersonal communication and the nurse-patient relationship. This will assist us in providing a more comprehensive explanation of the level of service that each individual patient can expect to receive.

So far, quality has been considered in the light of the nursing profession and how this may affect the patients' experience of the health-care service. The Patient's Charter states that one of the objectives of the document is to ensure that the patient is always put first and that the service provided produces clear, measurable benefits to the patient's health. Thus, quality in terms of the Patient's Charter must incorporate meeting the requirements of patients and, therefore, assumes a customer concern for the development and maintenance of high standards within the NHS.

To date, much of the literature concerning quality focuses on the professional needs and aspirations of developing services, with little more than lip service being paid to the role of the consumer. The inference, here, is that the health-care professional knows best. This may be true to some extent, but the one thing we all have in common with our patients is that we are also users, or prospective users, of health-care services. This suggests that we should work far more closely with our patients, ensuring that their views and opinions are actively incorporated into future plans and developments, in order to maintain a service that is responsive to people's views and needs.

Various approaches have been taken to develop the inclusion of consumer views. Initiatives that are currently being used are the monitoring and response of patient complaints, focused patient satisfaction surveys, the establishment of user groups and the use of open meetings. However, this seems a limited approach, considering the large number of consumers the NHS has. The majority of these initiatives are operating on an organisational level and do not, therefore, encapsulate the issues that perhaps appear small and less significant to an organisation but are of great importance to individual patients.

This can be highlighted from my own personal experience. I was recently admitted to a surgical ward for minor surgery. I was somewhat uncomfortable in what was a new role to me: that of a patient. I had received my premedication and was very sleepy when a porter and staff nurse lifted me from my bed and placed me on a trolley. As I was being wheeled down the corridor towards the operating theatre, the nurse in charge of the ward came running towards us shouting, 'Bring him back to the ward, they've got someone bleeding'. Following this incident, I was unable to consider the care I received during my stay in the same light. I could understand the reasons for bringing me back to the ward and could understand the necessity of the nurse informing her colleagues why I should go back to the ward. However, what remained with me was the way in which it was done. I began to question the confidentiality that surrounded my care and, more importantly to me as a person, the ability of the staff to deal with difficult or emergency situations. I also began to feel like a number on an operating list, a task to be performed, but a task that had to be delayed because of difficulties in completing a previous task.

This incident does not directly reflect the quality of the surgery I received, nor does it reflect the quality of the post-operative care I received. However, it did form a

large part of my overall perception of the quality of service
I experienced. It also stressed to me the importance of
actively encouraging patients to play their part in assessing
the quality of the service they receive, as the patient retains
a perspective very different from that of the nurse. It
also demonstrates the importance of nurses working in
collaboration with others involved in the health-care
service. The Patient's Charter identifies in national standard no. 2 that arrangements ensure that everyone can use
services, including people with special needs. It is perhaps
not the nurses' direct responsibility if some patients are
unable to access some services, but, within the spirit of
the Patient's Charter, nurses must accept the responsibility
of working with others to ensure that national standards
are achieved, in order to provide a quality of service
acceptable to patients. Difficulty in accessing a service will
surely be associated with the way in which nursing care is
provided, once patients are in a position to consider their
experience.

Quality, therefore, is not only an issue that health-care
workers are being asked to adopt as part of their practice,
but one that they should discuss in terms of ethics, rights,
duties and accountability. For nurses to do justice to both
the Charter and the service they provide, it is essential
that they look beyond establishing a definition for quality
or including a statement about it in their philosophy of
care. To ensure that the concept of quality is incorporated
into the nursing service and that effective quality assurance
programmes are developed, nurses need to examine every
aspect of their practice, especially the ethical dimension.
This includes not only the tasks that nurses perform and
the procedures they follow, but also the way in which
nurses do things, the overall perception of their service by
others — other health-care professionals and patients
alike — and the way in which nurses relate to the wider
society.

The standards within the Charter offer nurses a baseline for quality initiatives within their practice, but we now need to develop these further. It is not enough to monitor and develop the quality of service through professional and jargon-laden quality assurance programmes; nurses now need to encourage a more participative approach that enables both nurses and patients objectively to comment on the quality of nursing services and also on where nurses would like these services to be influential in the future.

In terms of ethics, these considerations can be summed up in the following points.

• Ethics is about acting with and towards people; the relationship between clients and professionals is, therefore, of paramount importance.
• The relationship is characterised by 'being' as well as 'doing', i.e. by enabling access to care at many levels as well as by direct care.
• How are nurses' perceptions of health care altered when they are recipients of care?
• Quality is about more than achieving certain standards; it is about treatment given with respect, rather than just a task performed.
• Conversely, ethics is not only about theoretical principles, but also about everyday activities, services and attitudes.

The Named Nurse

It would not be possible to discuss the nurse's view of the Patient's Charter without considering the named nurse concept. The Patient's Charter specifically identifies the nurse as an integral part of the initiative. National standard no. 8 states:

The Charter Standard is that you should have a named,

qualified nurse, midwife, or health visitor who will be responsible for your nursing or midwifery care.

This is, however, no new notion. Florence Nightingale (1869) described a similar method of caring for patients when she considered the case method of nursing patients. It is also true that many nurses have always worked in this way. For other nurses, however, the standard requires a rethink about the way in which nursing teams provide care and the role that each nurse takes within that team.

The identification of a single named nurse to organise and coordinate an individual's care does not automatically suggest that a primary nursing approach must be taken. Obviously, the organisation of care using primary nursing makes implementation of this standard far easier, but other methods that focus on the patient as an individual are easily adapted. Wright (1993) explores many of the questions that arise from this standard and identifies the different ways in which implementation can be effected in a variety of care settings. He identifies numerous approaches, for example patient allocation, team nursing, case management and key worker systems, that can effectively adopt the named nurse initiative.

It is not the Charter's intention to dictate how all nursing care should be delivered (for example as primary nursing), as this would only inhibit the development of new systems and models of nursing care delivery. It is the intention, however, to demonstrate the important role that nurses play within health care. The Charter recognises that nurses are the constant companions of patients throughout their health-care experience, whether in the community or in hospital.

Wright (1993) states that the spirit of named nursing is about providing a focal point to help guide the patient through the health-care system. As the focal point, the nurse assists in helping to resolve problems and works together with the patient, relatives, friends and other carers. This is an essential part of the standard, enabling the patient and significant others to identify a single nurse who can provide direct care and information about that care. The named nurse is also able to ensure continuity of care and act as an anchor point when the patient is confronted with a sea of busy health-care professionals. In this sense, the named nurse can be seen as the nursing team's representative to the patient.

However, the named nurse can also be seen as the patient's representative to the rest of the health-care team. The named nurse is able to participate in the development of comprehensive treatment programmes and ensure that the evaluation of the prescribed care is constantly taken back to the health-care team. This also establishes a route for patients to deliver their views and opinions of treatment and care to the health-care team.

This standard also gives the qualified nurse the responsibility for nursing care. Responsibilities are usually outlined in job descriptions, and the level of these responsibilities will normally be reflected in the grade of the post. They can be seen as the duties of that post, although Tschudin (1992) suggests that responsibility is a far wider concept than being just duty. On exploring the concept further, it is linked to freedom, goodness and rightness. However, Tschudin (1992) also states that to have responsibility means to respond, to answer to someone or something, and is, therefore, linked to accountability.

Within the Charter, qualified nurses have responsibility for nursing care. They must, therefore, respond to and answer patients. This suggests the free flow and exchange of information, which can only be achieved with the establishment of clearly defined channels of communication. With the implied closeness of this relationship, and responsibility going beyond duty, the nurse may well become concerned about becoming 'involved' with the patient. Tschudin (1992) believes that the nurse's role is to care, and not to become 'involved' is, perhaps, not to fulfil that role. The implication of the Charter is that nurses must become 'involved' with the patients they are responsible for, responding to and answering them.

Tschudin's (1992) thoughts and the implications of the Patient's Charter do not identify anything new to the nursing world. Peplau (1952) suggested that nurses could only work with the information that patients gave them. Clearly, patients are always providing nurses with some form of information, even if this is simply details about their immediate problems, for example a fractured limb demonstrated by X-ray. To meet the patient's needs effectively, the nurse must exchange information, develop channels of communication and become 'involved' with the patient, so that care is effective and of benefit to the patient.

The idea of developing channels of communication and becoming 'involved' with the patient is essential to the effective functioning of the named nurse. Gersie and King (1990) consider issues of storytelling that can be compared with the patient giving information to the nurse. The teller of the story, i.e. the patient, will usually have specific reasons for choosing to tell a particular story at a particular moment. It may be told to affect a decision or to safeguard some important issue. Gersie and King (1990) suggest that the teller may relate the story to purge, console, guide or instruct, which is relevant to the teller and listener alike. However, whatever the reason for telling the story, the result is that it provides meaning for both nurse and patient.

It is, therefore, important to recognise that developing channels of communication for information exchange not only facilitates the delivery of health care, but also provides meaning. By providing the means for patients to speak openly and freely, the named nurse is assisting patients to

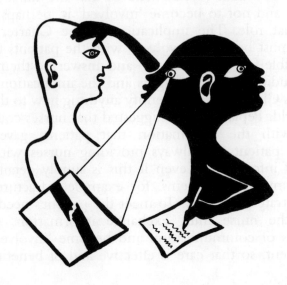

give meaning and understanding to their health status and recognising them as individuals, thus adapting their care accordingly.

The inextricable link between responsibility and accountability is also identified by Manley (1991), who believes that accountability is part of being professional. This idea is supported by Denyes et al (1989), who suggest that scientific accountability is a characteristic of a profession. Leddy and Pepper (1989) take the notion one step further and state that the concept of the professional includes both legal and moral accountability for the individual's own actions. Burnard and Chapman (1988) suggest that being accountable is not only answering for one's practice, but also understanding its origins and the powers of carrying it out. Alternatively, as Marks-Maran (1993) believes, 'accountability is justifying actions by understand-

ing the rationale behind them and the possible consequences of such actions'.

The question then arises of whether the nurse who is
responsible is also accountable. The simplest way to consider this is, perhaps, that responsibility can be delegated
and accountability cannot. A request to a junior nurse to
perform a task, for example, is asking her or him to accept
responsibility for that task. The nurse's responsibility is to
do the job to the best of their ability, to do a good job
and to do it correctly. However, the senior nurse will
retain the accountability for that task in that she or he is
answerable for it being performed to an acceptable level,
that the nurse actually doing it is capable of doing so
and that the senior nurse understands the rationale for that
task and can make an informed decision about it (Marks-
Maran, 1993).

Informed decision-making in the context of nursing
practice suggests that nurses must be able to change the
direction of care-giving based on their knowledge of
the situation. To be truly responsible and accountable for
their practice, nurses must, therefore, also have the authority to make decisions about the care they deliver. This
dismisses the myth that the sister/charge nurse knows best
for all patients. It requires each and every qualified nurse
to function as an individual practitioner. However, no
single health-care professional can meet all the needs of
any one patient. To do so would be putting the patient at
risk, and, as such, to work as an individual practitioner does
not mean working in isolation. Individual practitioners are
able to make decisions about the direction of care, ensuring
that any change incorporates the overall views of the
health-care team they represent.

This, in turn, clearly demonstrates the importance that
the Charter places on the role of the nurse within the
health-care team. Qualified nurses are answerable for their
practice to clients, other members of the health-care team

and the rest of the profession. This is a public declaration of nurses' importance in health care, and, as such, nurses need to 'stand up and be counted' for their practice. Nurses are not only 'counted' in this initiative but also named. This means that the named nurse is a very public figure — a nurse who is known by patients and carers alike and must, therefore, be confident and competent in her or his practice.

This is clearly a great demand placed on all qualified nurses. Purely having undergone a period of education, which has led to nurse registration, does not mean that all newly registered nurses are able to meet the demands implicit in the named nurse standard of the Charter. The nuances involved in adapting to working as a registered nurse are numerous and varied, and, as such, newly qualified nurses need time to adapt to their change in role. To be asked to function as a named nurse, with all its responsibilities, will not enable the initiative to flourish for the individual nurse, the nursing profession or the patient. Nurses must be given the opportunity to develop in this role to ensure appropriate fulfilment.

It would not seem appropriate to identify specific educational routes for this development to take. Nurses who are moving towards taking on the role of the named nurse will have different skills, knowledge, abilities and experiences, all of which need to be acknowledged. Learning needs to take on an individual quality, each nurse identifying his or her own educational needs, in conjunction with a mentor or supervisor, and moving towards agreed objectives. This enables individual nurses to develop at a pace that they dictate. Thus, when taking on the role of the named nurse, they are confident and competent in their abilities and offer a secure and trusting environment for the patient.

If many qualified nurses are to take on these responsibilities, what then happens to the role of the sister/charge

nurse? Earlier, it was suggested that the myth of sister/
charge nurse knowing best could be dismissed. This is
perhaps not entirely true. It is certainly no longer appropriate for the sister/charge nurse to know every single detail
about all the patients: their age, diagnosis, current treatment, care plans, etc. However, the focus of the role has
changed in the light of the named nurse initiative within
the Charter. Sisters/charge nurses now need to take on
more of a coordinating role, ensuring that all patients have
a named nurse and that individual nurses are able to fulfil
their roles appropriately. The sister/charge nurse now
needs to act as an informed advisor, not only where clinical
tasks and procedures are concerned, but also in role development. The role of the sister/charge nurse as mentor is
essential to ensure the development of both nurses and
nursing practice. It is perhaps more appropriate now to
see these senior nurses as individuals who control the care
environment and ensure that it is appropriate to the needs
of the patient group, and who act as role models and are
catalysts for practice development.

The named nurse standard, therefore, goes further than
offering patients the name of a nurse for the duration of
their health-care episode. It endeavours to take individual-
ised patient care further, by offering patients a pathway for
participating in the development and delivery of their
health care. The implications for nurses are far-reaching.
The named nurse concept recognises the valuable contribution that nurses make to health-care delivery, but, more
than that, it requires nurses constantly to reflect on their
interactions and interventions with patients, their role
within the health-care team, their own development and
education and their ethical stance. It forces nurses to
review their roles within nursing teams and to develop
new ones to meet the changing needs of patients and
service delivery. This standard requires nurses to review
the levels to which they are responsible and accountable

for their practice and to continue the development of professionalism within nursing.

The ethical issues discussed in this section can be highlighted as the following:

- The named nurse concept asks for a re-evaluation of the issues of responsibility and accountability.
- The named nurse idea gives patients a right and carers a corresponding responsibility.
- Issues such as 'involvement' and 'meaning' take on new importance in the overall care of the patient.
- Education, learning needs, control of care environments and the participation in and development of health-care delivery need to be seen in terms of ethics and ethical behaviour towards patients as individuals and towards society as a whole.

The Individual Nurse

As discussed earlier, not all nurses work as named nurses, and the implications of the Charter for them must also be explored.

The need to work with our patients and to ensure that the rights and standards of the Charter are achieved applies to all nurses. Wright (1994) believes that the Charter is a test for nurses. It is an opportunity for nurses to review their commitment to advocacy and empowering patients and to negotiate and work in partnership with patients, as opposed to exercising power over them.

Power can be seen as two distinct areas: 'power over' and 'power to'. 'Power over' has been described by Hokanson Hawks (1991) as the ability to influence the behaviour and decisions of others to obey or conform. This concept has a directive force or impact and suggests a struggle for dominance, encompassing control, competitiveness and authority. This is obviously at odds with the Patient's Charter, in which the objective is to provide patients with more information, a monitoring tool for service provision and a more active role in health care.

King (1981) believes power to be goal-directed, involving human interaction and being the actual or potential ability or capacity to achieve goals. Supporting this notion, Hokanson Hawks (1991) suggests that 'power to' is the actual or potential ability or capacity to achieve objectives through an interpersonal process in which the goals and the means to achieve these goals are mutually agreed and worked towards. She believes that, in order to achieve this, there must be antecedents of self-confidence, power skills such as trust, communication skills, knowledge, concern, respect and caring. All these have already been identified as necessities for the development of a quality and ethical nursing service in response to the Patient's Charter.

Raatikainen (1994) considers power within nursing care and suggests that powerful people are intellectual and creative and have a good self-image. She also believes that they are internally motivated, have clear values, respect others and have a well-developed ability to collaborate with others. Although Raatikainen's (1994) observations are related to nurses, it appears evident that in order for patients to be powerful individuals, they too must possess these qualities. The Patient's Charter, therefore, necessitates the development of powerful people or the empowerment of nurses and patients alike.

In nursing literature generally and in the process of implementing new initiatives within the NHS, there has been an increasing use of the term 'empowerment'. However, there is little within the clinical environment, whether in the community or in institutions, to assist nurses in understanding the concept or how to develop it practically. Gibson (1991) suggests that 'empowerment' refers to inequalities of power between individuals and between different layers of society. She suggests that the concept is used within everyday nursing practice and that questions should be asked about social and economic factors that influence good health. Perhaps the most fundamental and unarticulated statement within the Patient's Charter is about 'empowerment' — the empowerment of patients to reduce the unequal distribution of power and to develop a more equitable uptake of services, thus having the potential to influence their health status.

However, as Skelton (1994) asserts, empowerment is not about maintaining the idea that the professional knows best and getting the patient to come round to the professional's point of view, which the nurse asserts in advance to be best for the patient. When interpreting empowerment as the handing over of power in relation to health care, nurses must accept that theirs is not the only way to proceed. Here, we see the importance of the collaborative approach to care and negotiating the way forward. What empowerment introduces is the notion of compromise. That is not to say that nurses should put the patient at risk by compromising safety, but rather that they should accommodate the patient's wishes within the provision of health care. For example, in order to meet patients' personal hygiene needs, nurses often make efforts to ensure that patients are bathed on a regular basis. However, this is possibly meeting the needs of nurses more than patients, and nurses may be seen to be imposing their own views of personal hygiene on the patient. In some instances, patients may never bathe, perhaps because they are not used to it or because of physical difficulties in actually bathing themselves. It is at this point that nurses will need to compromise to accommodate the patient's wishes not to bathe at all but to have regular all-over washes.

Skelton (1994) believes that empowerment should be considered on both a micro and a macro level. The micro level is perhaps the most significant for nurses, who, as

Malin and Teasdale (1991) suggest, put their skills and knowledge at the disposal of the patient, who is trusted to make responsible decisions. At a macro level, empowerment concerns the organisation and management levels, in that decisions regarding health-care services incorporate patients' needs, views and opinions. From the patients' perspective, there is certainly ample room for a redistribution of power, nurses devolving some degree of responsibility to patients and thus reducing some of the dependency on the providers (Skelton, 1994). At a macro level, this will necessitate that managers of organisations recognise the collective voice of patients and act on it, whether this voice is represented by patients themselves or by nurses as their representatives.

If one considers empowerment to be one of the main thrusts of the Patient's Charter, it must be clearly defined in order to be appropriately effected. It is unlikely that there will be a shift of resources to those who are currently disempowered, and the nurses' aim must, therefore, be to encourage consultation and discussion on service delivery and ensure that representation of nurses and patients exists in decision-making forums. This needs to be applied at both macro and micro levels, for individual patient care and the overall provision of health-care services. The concept of empowerment within the Patient's Charter will almost certainly mean that nurses must take on an advocacy role. However, more importantly, in putting the concept of empowerment into practice, nurses are demonstrating a commitment to working with their patients in a concerted effort to change the way in which health care is currently provided. As such, nurses are working towards achieving one of the overall objectives of the Patient's Charter in improving and modernising the delivery of health-care services.

It does not appear possible to discuss empowerment without considering advocacy and the nurse's role as the patient's advocate. Marks–Maran (1993) considers advocacy from different perspectives and offers arguments both for and against the concept. She suggests that nurses are seeking to decide whether or not there is a role for them as advocates and, if there is, what that role should be. In making these decisions, Marks–Maran (1993) believes that nursing should take perspectives alternative to those of the legal definitions offered and begin to explore the issues within a total value system of caring.

When considering a total value system, we cannot afford to focus purely on the value systems of each individual nurse. Consideration needs to be given to the value system of the organisation within which nurses work and the forces that are driving it. In this way, the Patient's Charter becomes incorporated into the nurses' value system as a driving force of the NHS. As such, nurses cannot afford to ignore the initiatives identified within it, in particular the drive to empower patients through participation in monitoring the service, the identification of choice and the provision of accurate information about the services that are provided. This makes it impossible to dismiss the notion of nurses acting as the patients' advocate. In turn, this makes it necessary to modify the available definitions identifying the extent to which nurses are able to fulfil this role.

Nelson (1988) suggests that advocacy has always been a part of nursing but that, in practical terms, nurses have progressed from a position of acting as mediators. Nurses now act as supporters of patients. Especially in situations in which patients are not present, they act as guardians of patients' rights to autonomy and informed choice. Advocacy can thus be seen as a way of assisting patients in moving towards and establishing independence. How this is achieved must, however, be carefully considered. In representing patients and pleading their cases for them without ensuring that they have all the relevant information, nurses can, arguably, be seen as making patients passive and, in the extreme, as manipulating patients' opportunity for choice in order to meet their own needs. One of the overall aims of the Charter is to transform patients from passive recipients of care to active individuals in the health-care process. If we define advocacy inaccurately and act on that wrong definition, we are in danger of ignoring a major aspect of the Patient's Charter.

Ersser and Tutton (1991) suggest that part of the process of advocacy for nurses is to ensure that there are sufficient resources for patients, in order that rights are upheld. However, if nurses lack confidence in their ability and do not possess the necessary authority and power, their role as advocates will have no meaning when decisions made with the patient conflict with those made by other members of the health-care team. It is all too easy to complain about the lack of resources and, therefore, the inability to maintain a role as the patients' advocate. In these instances, a wider, more encompassing approach needs to be taken. Nurses have control over a number of resources, which should not be seen purely as the equipment or finance available to provide a service. Although improvements in both these areas can make life easier, they do not necessarily increase the quality of the service available. Nurses should view their time, skills and knowledge and the information they can offer as a resource and, as such, are able to uphold many of the patients' rights without entering into conflict with others.

The Patient's Charter provides nurses with the authority and power necessary to develop the role of patient advocate. The named nurse standard states the responsibility of the nurse and, as such, it is for nurses to decide how this can best be achieved. Nurses are in a position to have detailed knowledge of patients and their viewpoint. They have direct communication with other members of the health-care team, and the Charter provides them with

the vehicle to establish sufficient authority to challenge
any decision that is believed to impinge on patients' rights
or to support patients in their decisions regarding their
health and health care.

The giving and receiving of information has featured
throughout this discussion, particularly in relation to
empowerment and advocacy. In order to encourage
patients to work towards independence and make
informed decisions about their care, nurses need to provide
information truthfully and in a way that allows patients a
complete understanding. Tschudin (1993) suggests that it
is appropriate for nurses to play an increasingly active part
in informing patients, as nurses generally spend more time
with patients. She believes that nurses are in a better
position to know their patients' characters and can relate
to patients informally and discuss issues as an integral part
of caring. Sadly, a recent Royal College of Nursing report
(RCN, 1994) finds that most people have limited knowledge about their rights under the Patient's Charter and
stresses that patients cannot exercise their rights unless they
are better informed about them. The need for explicit
information is essential to encourage a participative
approach in direct health care and the development of
health-care services.

Herriott and Morris (1994) believe this situation to be
indicative of a lack of communication between nurses and
patients. This may be so, but nurses must also consider the
nature of the information that they provide and whether
or not patients are able to assimilate that information.
Providing written information or giving a rehearsed dia-
logue may still not improve this situation. Information as
important as that which relates to our health, or the service
we receive in relation to our health, must be understandable. Too much jargon-laden literature can be as ineffective
as providing no information at all. Information is an integral part of communication skills, and nurses must find

suitable methods of providing this. Whether it is in speech or in writing, it needs to be short, simple, free from jargon and explicit (Tschudin, 1993).

As individual nurses take on the roles of empowering patients and acting as their advocates, they are developing current nursing practice and changing the way in which nurses traditionally function. As such, nurses must be seen as change agents within the health-care environment. Most health-care providers are seen as highly complex organisations to which change does not come easily. Many nurses' past experiences have resulted in frustration when attempts have been made to bring about changes to improve and facilitate everyday health-care delivery.

However, the Patient's Charter can, in itself, be seen as a change agent, thus providing nurses with the opportunity of bringing about changes as part of its implementation. When examining change, the organisation within which each nurse works can be considered as a microcosm of society itself. The members of that society, or employees, construct a reality according to the norms and values, or culture, of that organisation. In such an organisation, the behaviour of individuals is consistent with the reality that has been created (Ellis and Whittington, 1993). Thus, the behaviour of nurses conforms to that which is acceptable to and requested by the organisation. The culture of the organisation is demonstrated through the formal and informal structures, systems and hierarchies and the way in which communication networks are organised. The introduction of a new approach, or of change, will only be successful if it conforms to the recognised norms and values of the organisation.

Change, therefore, can be seen as an uphill struggle within the complexities of health-care organisations. However, with the Charter's message of working in collaboration with patients, nurses can effectively work with, and on behalf of, patients to focus the norms and values of the organisation on a patient-centred approach to health care. This can be done in a localised way, when working directly with patients through the health-care team, and in a global way, by ensuring nurse representation in strategic service planning and development forums.

Much of this may sound like idealism. However, Ottaway (1982) identifies a change strategy that focuses on change as a social process, and this, after all, is what the Patient's Charter is about: patients changing from being passive receivers of health care to being active participants in achieving and maintaining optimum health status. The Charter is aiming to change the way in which society views and receives health-care services. Johns (1991) suggests that one of the reasons why change agents need to come from within the change environment is that they have legitimate authority to make the change. The Patient's Charter has provided nurses with that legitimate authority by introducing the named nurse standard.

Within the changing environment, the sister/charge nurse must again take on the role of supervisor and mentor. Mason et al (1990) describe how nurses can be empowered to make changes through an education programme. Change, however, is not a process that will occur overnight, particularly where norms and values need to be further developed, so focusing purely on an education programme will not achieve the necessary forward movement. The role of the sister/charge nurse as mentor is essential to maintain the commitment and motivation for change, to create the opportunities for discussion, to raise awareness in all forums of the key issues and to provide the personal and technical support necessary for the changes to be effected. This also requires a commitment from managers to ensure observation, supervision and evaluation of changed behaviour. Change agents are, therefore, powerful people, both up and down hierarchies and diagonally across to colleagues and clients.

For nurses to act as effective change agents, and for the delivery of health care to make the major shift towards collaborative, patient-focused care, the way in which it is organised must be given careful consideration. It is impractical to attempt to make such a change over a short period of time, especially when it is likely that there will need to be a change in norms and values, some of which will be so subtle that they may be difficult to identify. To some extent, the Patient's Charter has shown a way forward for that change by identifying a number of national Charter standards, which nurses should work towards achieving but not expect to attain immediately. To act as change agents, nurses need to work together in an organised fashion, thus preventing results from being haphazard and inconsistent. Unfortunately, there is no single formula to follow, as the design of change is unique to each setting (Johns, 1991); as such, nurses must use their skills and the relationships they have with their patients to assist them in this process.

It is evident from this discussion that all nurses have a large part to play in relation to the Patient's Charter. Not all nurses will function as named nurses, but this does not mean that there is no role for them within the Charter. It is also evident that although some of the issues identified are complex, their implementation and development cannot be left only to the most senior nurses. All nurses can, and must, work towards the development of their role and the delivery of health care. Only in taking on their role as professionals, i.e. acting ethically, can nurses change and influence. The Charter gives them a start, but nurses have to commit themselves, both individually and as a profession, to be seen to be ethical.

The ethical issues discussed under the heading of 'The Individual Nurse' are the following:

- Empowering patients creates a more equal and just society, justice being an essential aspect of health care.
- The role of patient advocate has to be considered carefully by nurses as an essential part of empowerment.
- Social and economic factors influence good health; how can they be distributed more equally?
- Autonomy and informed choice are basic necessities of decision-making; how can advocacy foster them?
- Information and truth are pillars of patient care; how do nurses foster both?

Conclusion

In order to introduce these essential changes in practice it is easy to offer suggestions that follow the accepted route, by calling for nurse educators to take a leading role, as nurses cannot be expected to take on new roles if they are not adequately educated to do so. However, although input from educators is necessary, this is not the most important factor in the successful implementation of the Patient's Charter. The most pressing implication for nurses that can be taken from the Charter is the change in nature of health-care provision and the essential change in culture within health-care organisations.

The Charter is instrumental in moving health-care services further towards a market economy and, as such, is using methods similar to those of other markets to monitor and develop service provision. The Charter is asking its users, both purchasers and patients, to comment on and become involved in the standards to which the service operates. Nurses need to be involved at two levels: at the level of strategic planning within management structures and at a clinical level, where they are constantly in touch with the users of services. There is, therefore, a role

for all nurses within the Patient's Charter, regardless of
grade or perceived importance within the nursing hierarchy. This is further accentuated when the culture of
organisations is considered. Nurses are the constant companions of patients during their health-care episode and,
as such, must constantly represent them and their views,
continuing to remind the health-care team that patients
are the focus of care and treatment and steer it back
towards them.

It is necessary for nurses to work more closely with
others, not just other members of the health-care team,
but all members of the organisation who work towards
enhancing the service. Health-care provision has seen the
introduction of general managers, administrators and business managers, and it is working together that will enhance
health-care delivery and achieve the rights and standards
that are clearly set out in the Patient's Charter.

I recall a meeting I attended recently at which it was
explicitly stated that nurses were totally responsible for the
effective implementation of the Patient's Charter. I dispute
this. Nurses certainly have a major role to play and are
identified as professionals who have an important part to
play in the development of health-care delivery. They are,
however, unable to perform this task alone and, as such,
cannot, and should not, accept total responsibility for it.
The responsibility of each individual nurse is to fulfil his
or her identified role, whether explicit or implicit, and to
encourage and support others in doing the same.

However, to incorporate the concepts identified within
this chapter into everyday practice necessitates a change of
the nurse's role. It is no longer possible to cling to tra-
ditional roles and it is apparent that there is a dichotomy
between the essentials of being a good nurse and those of
good nursing practice. Taylor (1992) suggests that patients
value the human element of nurses, i.e. the caring and
interactive characteristics. Good nurses also need to have

a sound knowledge base and the ability to perform clinical skills expertly. To respond effectively to the demands of the Patient's Charter, nursing needs to work with both areas. Nurses' knowledge base and clinical skills must continue to be a demonstrable asset, but far more emphasis needs to be placed on the value of the therapeutic relationship, and more research has to be undertaken to demonstrate the benefits of this aspect of the nursing role.

Many readers will assert that the patient has always been the focus of nursing and that knowledge, skills and interaction have always been considered. This is, to some extent, true, but the Patient's Charter is requesting that the patient is viewed in a different light and now becomes an active focus rather than purely the recipient of care and treatment. It seems necessary, therefore, that in the acquisition of knowledge and skills, nurses should ensure that the therapeutic relationship becomes an integral part of all aspects of nursing and ceases to be considered in isolation. Only when that relationship itself is considered ethically important can change occur where it is needed, i.e. in the actual delivery of care.

The Patient's Charter has numerous implications for nurses and nursing. It empowers nurses and offers them the opportunity to strengthen their position within health-care teams and develop the nursing profession. More than this, it focuses health care and treatment on the individual patients, which necessitates constant reflection and evaluation of the services that nurses provide. These services are also increasingly seen as being given ethically.

References

Avis M (1992) Consumer cures. *Senior Nurse*, 12(5), pp. 5–8.
Barber P (1991) Caring — the nature of a therapeutic relation-

ship. In Perry A and Jolley M (eds), *Nursing: A Knowledge Base for Practice*. London: Edward Arnold, pp. 230–70.

Burnard P and Chapman C (1988) *Professional and Ethical Issues in Nursing, The Code of Professional Conduct*. Chichester: John Wiley.

Denyes M J, Connor N A, Oakley D and Ferguson S (1989) Integrating nursing theory, practice and research through collaborative research. *Journal of Advanced Nursing*, 14(2), pp. 141–5.

DoH (Department of Health) (1989) *Working for Patients*. London: HMSO.

DoH (Department of Health) (1991) *The Patient's Charter*. London: HMSO.

Ellis R (ed.) (1988) *Professional Competence and Quality Assurance in the Caring Professions*. London: Croom Helm.

Ellis R and Whittington D (1993) *Quality Assurance In Health Care, A Handbook*. London: Edward Arnold.

Ersser R and Tutton E (eds) (1991) *Primary Nursing in Perspective*. London: Scutari Press.

Gersie A and King N (1990) *Storymaking in education and therapy*. London: Jessica Kingsley.

Gibson C (1991) A concept analysis of empowerment. *Journal of Advanced Nursing*, 16(3), pp. 354–61.

Hokanson Hawks J (1991) Power: a concept analysis. *Journal of Advanced Nursing*, 16(6), pp. 754–62.

Herriott S and Morris M (1994) RCN report highlights the limitations of The Patient's Charter. *British Journal of Nursing*, 3(9), pp. 440–1.

Johns C (1991) Introducing and managing change — the move to primary nursing. In Ersser R and Tutton E (eds), *Primary Nursing in Perspective*. London: Scutari Press, pp. 31–47.

King I (1981) *A Theory for Nursing. Systems, Concepts, Process*. New York: John Wiley.

Leddy S and Pepper J M (1989) *Conceptual Bases of Professional Nursing*. Philadelphia: J B Lippincott.

Malin N and Teasdale K (1991) Caring versus empowerment: considerations for nursing practice. *Journal of Advanced Nursing*, 16(6), pp. 657–62.

Manley K (1991) Knowledge for nursing practice. In Perry A

and Jolley M (eds), *Nursing: A Knowledge Base for Practice.* London: Edward Arnold, pp. 1–27.

Marks-Maran D (1993) Advocacy. In Tschudin V (ed.), *Ethics: Nurses and Patients.* London: Scutari Press, pp. 65–83.

Mason D J, Costello-Nickitas D M, Scanlon J M and Magnuson B A (1990) Empowering nurses for politically astute change in the workplace. *Journal of Continuing Education in Nursing,* 22(1), pp. 5–10.

Nelson M L (1988) Advocacy in nursing. *Nursing Outlook,* 36(3), pp. 136–41.

Nightingale F (1869) *Notes on Nursing, What It Is and What It Is Not.* Republished 1980. Edinburgh: Churchill Livingstone.

Ottaway R M (1982) Defining the change agent. In Evans B, Powell J A and Talbot F (eds), *Changing Design.* Chichester: John Wiley.

Peplau H (1952) *Interpersonal Relations in Nursing.* New York: Putnam.

Raatikainen R (1994) Power or the lack of it in nursing care. *Journal of Advanced Nursing,* 19(3), pp. 424–32.

RCN (Royal College of Nursing) (1994) *Unchartered Territory: Public Awareness of The Patient's Charter.* London: RCN.

Skelton R (1994) Nursing and empowerment: concepts and strategies. *Journal of Advanced Nursing,* 19(3), pp. 415–23.

Taylor B J (1992) From helper to human: a reconceptualisation of the nurse as a person. *Journal of Advanced Nursing,* 17(9), pp. 1042–4.

Tschudin V (1992) *Ethics in Nursing, The Caring Relationship* (2nd edn). Oxford: Butterworth-Heinemann.

Tschudin V (ed.) (1993) *Ethics: Nurses and Patients.* London: Scutari Press.

Wilson-Barnett J (1981) Janforum. *Journal of Advanced Nursing,* 6(6), pp. 503–14.

Wright S (ed.) (1993) *The Named Nurse, Midwife and Health Visitor.* London: NHSME Department of Health, HMSO.

Wright S (1994) Turn tables on 'top down' Tories. *Nursing Standard,* 8(33), p. 35.

CHAPTER 2

A Doctor's View

Peter Baddeley

This chapter has been written by a GP with many years of experience caring for people. He writes as someone who looks at the Patient's Charter from a practical point of view: how do the various rights and standards affect GPs and patients in practical terms?

The author presents himself to readers like a good chairperson: stating many facts and then inviting debate on the ethics behind the facts. The questions at the end of each section point to the general problem of the ethics surrounding the Patient's Charter, namely the rights and responsibilities of patients and carers, providers and purchasers. Doubts are raised and problems uncovered, and readers are invited to formulate their own questions, too, in order to widen the discussion still further.

The philosopher Wilhelm Reich states radically and forcefully that 'the physician or teacher has only one obligation, that of practising his profession uncompromisingly . . . and to consider only the welfare of those who are given into his care' (Reich, 1940). In other words, physicians, surgeons, nurses, and any other health professionals have only one duty, which is to place the needs of their patients before all other considerations. By virtue of our vocation and training, we profess to know what is required for our patients and the most appropriate way of meeting those needs. If professionalism were so enlightened, patients would have no need of any Charter, but the realities of life are more complex.

The consultation between physician and patient is not sacrosanct. Doctors are aware of the constraints of time (the 12 further patients to be seen in the clinic), material resources (for example, the number of dialysis machines or donor kidneys available for transplant) and financial resources (the comparative cost of drugs of varying efficacy and with differing degrees of adverse effect). There are two other important areas that Reich's exhortation omits. We have a duty to learn from those under our care and, by research, improve medical, surgical and nursing procedures. We also should extend our responsibility to the patients of the future by training new members of our own and associated professions.

As health-care professionals, our first obligation remains to the individual patient in our care, but it is not our sole obligation. Even that primary obligation is compromised by many other considerations and some factors beyond our control. Perhaps a Charter setting down what patients should expect from health-care professionals is not such a bad idea after all.

Charters have a long history. In the political context, they comprise a document or Bill of Rights conferred on the general population by a governing body. The Magna Carta, forced on King John in 1215, has become the cornerstone of the English Constitution. Attempts to build on this in the early 19th century (the People's Charter) and more recently (Charter 88) have not been as successful. We should, in principle therefore, welcome the recent introduction of a Citizen's and a Patient's Charter. There could, however, be difficulties when the rights and standards laid down in a Charter by government raise expectations in patients that are either incompatible with professional ethics or cannot be met by doctors and nurses employed by the government, yet who are professionally independent of government control.

If recent health service reforms were a complete success, we should not need a Charter at all. Until recently, the NHS was seen as a populist rather than a governmental

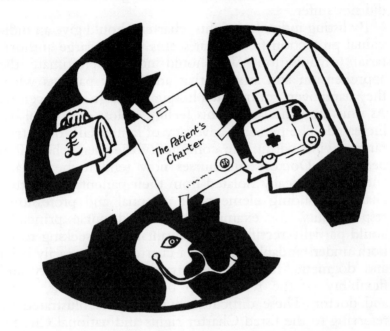

organisation. It was 'our doctor', 'our hospital' and 'our health service'. It could be said that the politicisation of the NHS and its fragmentation into purchasing and provider units, operating on a more commercial basis, has diminished this sense of ownership and led to the need for a written Charter.

The common ownership and cooperative nature of the NHS has its foundations in the utilitarian movement espoused by Jeremy Bentham and John Stuart Mill in the early 19th century. The essential doctrine of utilitarianism is that the right and ethical course of action is that which does the greatest good for the greatest number of people. The utilitarian movement was not repressive of individualism, and Mill, in particular, wrote passionately in defence of liberty and on the autonomy of the individual to do as he or she wished, providing that the rights of the majority did not suffer.

By listing individual rights, charters should give an individual protection from what seems to be a large authoritarian organisation. We should not underestimate the apprehension and anxiety that are felt by patients when they hand over 'control' at a hospital or large health centre. As units become larger, this feeling of loss of control has increased. The personal advocacy of family GPs or district nurses living within the community they serve has often been lost. Doctors and nurses now tend to be socially and geographically isolated from their patients. A written charter including elements of personal and professional responsibility, for example the named nurse principle, could partially rectify this disadvantage. By seeking to be both understandable and fair, a charter is necessarily brief and dogmatic. It can never match the complexity and flexibility of the relationship between a patient, nurse and doctor. These difficulties will now be illustrated by referring to the listed Charter rights and national Charter standards of the Patient's Charter (DoH, 1991).

The Existing Patient's Charter Rights

1. To receive health care on the basis of clinical need, regardless of ability to pay

The obligation to provide a comprehensive health service rests with the Secretary of State for Health, whose obligations in this respect are listed under Part 1 of the National Health Service Act 1977. Most of this act is still extant, although it has been considerably amended by subsequent legislation, particularly by the National Health Service and Community Care Act 1990. It is ethical that health care should be provided on the basis of clinical need; the legislation however makes specific exception for the recovery of charges. The Charter relates the commitment to providing comprehensive or even satisfactory health-care provision. Such definitions are hard to make and difficult to uphold. The scope and quality of health-care provision is linked to the financial and human resources available to the health service. It is the Secretary of State's responsibility to obtain sufficient resources from the Treasury in order to run the service. These resources have not always been forthcoming in the past. Many health service units have equipment funded, at least partly, by charitable appeals. Patients with a very rare or very serious illness often figure in media appeals for funds to enable them to travel abroad for treatment at some centre of excellence. Should we encourage our patients to lodge a complaint with purchaser units if they have to make use of equipment or services funded by charity rather than the State?

The NHS has long ceased to be totally free of charge. Fees for sight testing and dental work have been added to ever-increasing prescription charges, and this is allowed for in legislation. Those of our patients who do not have the ability to pay are asked to claim reimbursement or exemption, on appropriate forms. Thus, no-one is denied health care because of an inability to pay. However, there are difficulties. Provision of residential care for the elderly and disabled is a duty of Social Services departments administered by local authorities, and a contribution towards the cost of this social provision is expected. Long-term hospital care was, however, the provision of the NHS, and no charge was made for this. Since the early 1980s, many long-stay health service beds have been closed, and there has been a corresponding increase in the number of private sector nursing home beds. Patients needing long-term nursing care are still the responsibility of the NHS and the Secretary of State for Health. Patients discharged from hospital to a nursing home should, therefore, be funded by the health service, and, in theory at least, no contribution should be expected from the patient or family. This has not always happened, and test cases have been brought in the law courts. Judgement has reinforced the statutory obligation of the Secretary of State to provide nursing services free of charge, regardless of the ability to pay, but it seems odd that verification of the first Charter right has had to be sought through the courts.

• How ethical can health care be when the need for care has to be legally established?

2. To be registered with a GP

General medical practitioners operate independently of the NHS. This seems to have been forgotten by the general public, many health service administrators and even GPs themselves. There was intense discussion within the medical profession prior to the setting up of the NHS in 1948. It was felt that if GPs became a salaried part of the health service, as their hospital colleagues were, patients would have no independent advocate to whom they could turn. A compromise was reached. Patient and GP would sign an individual contract, but that contract would be administered by a third party, the Executive Council. Executive Councils have, in turn, been replaced by, Family Practitioner Committees (FPCs) and Family Health Service Authorities (FHSAs). This personal contract between doctor and patient led to GPs being thought of as 'my doctor' or even 'my private doctor', rather than 'the doctor' or 'the GP'. This close bond was furthered by the Medical Practices Committee. In order to encourage equity, the number and distribution of GPs was rigidly controlled by this Committee. Until recently, the chair and six of the other eight committee members had to be appointed from within the profession by the Secretary of State for Health. In essence, therefore, GPs themselves controlled the provision of GP services within the UK. Restricting the number of GP principals ensured equity of access, an even distribution of services and a reduction of waste through competition and avoidance of duplication. This has also, particularly in rural areas, reduced patient choice. Fortunately, this restriction has not caused disquiet, as the standard of general medical services is high. However, there are concerns for the future. The changes to the GP contract in 1990 angered many members of the profession. Some have retired early, recruitment has fallen and the morale in those who remain has plummeted. General medical practitioners, unlike their dental colleagues, have not resigned *en masse* from their NHS contracts. The legal right to be registered with and receive treatment from a general dental practitioner is not listed in the Patient's Charter. This omission might lead our patients to believe that this fundamental right no longer exists, and could be regarded as an ominous development.

• Should health services only exist in the presence of legal contracts?

3. To receive emergency medical care at any time, through your GP or the emergency ambulance service and hospital Accident & Emergency departments

A list of Charter rights may raise expectations. GPs are both contractually and professionally obliged to respond to medical emergencies, whether or not the patient is registered with them or their practice. Hospital Accident & Emergency departments and the ambulance service have similar obligations to treat genuine accidents and emergencies. The Charter does not mention that GPs have other obligations during their normal working week, as well as attending to accidents and emergencies at nights and weekends. Increasing patient demand, perhaps fuelled by the Patient's Charter, has led family doctors to call for an end to this 24-hour obligation. They are concerned not only for their own workload, but also for the effect of over-commitment on professional standards. It is not unusual for GPs to start work soon after 8 am in the morning, work throughout the day to the end of evening surgery at 6.30 pm and then do urgent and emergency visits until very late in the evening. They may then be called out of bed in the small hours and again at 6 am. Despite such a busy night on call, GPs will have to contend with another 8 am to 6.30 pm working day before they have a night off duty. Most GPs do a 34-hour stint at least once during each working week, and experience shows that many GPs work an average 54-hour week, excluding time spent on call.

Accident & Emergency departments have also become much busier. Many patients present with complaints of a relatively trivial nature. They attend because it is perceived to be more convenient than going to their GP, they do not want to 'worry' their GP or they may have been denied an appointment with their GP. A few patients attend because of dissatisfaction with the advice they have already been given by their GP. They want an immediate second opinion. Accident departments have become so concerned about this increase in expectation that some of them employ GPs on a sessional contract to treat and re-educate patients.

• Giving rights to one section of the population means exacting responsibilities from another section. Should such responsibilities be limitless?

4. To be referred to a consultant, acceptable to you, when your GP thinks it necessary, and to be referred for a second opinion if you and your GP agree this is desirable

The GP acts as a necessary 'gatekeeper' to the provision of secondary services, a situation that is peculiar to the UK. In many parts of Europe, patients can self-refer to specialists. The British method of referral reduces the cost of provision and the number of specialists required. It should also mean that patients are referred more appropriately. The wording of this Charter right reaffirms that referral is at the GP's discretion. Until recently, there was virtually no disincentive for GPs to refer patients who either did not respond to treatment or who seemed dissatisfied with the treatment given by the GP. Even so, failure to refer has often provoked complaints to FHSAs and litigation in the courts.

In theory, general practice fund holding should not act as a disincentive. GPs have been given the funds in order that they can make appropriate referrals to secondary providers quickly and efficiently. These funds are, however, limited, and fund-holding GPs now have to operate within financial constraints. There is now a disincentive to refer if the reason for referral seems doubtful or if GPs themselves feel that they can provide the service more cheaply 'in house'.

If GPs have chosen the correct specialist to see a patient, a second opinion should not be necessary. Occasionally, the problem is so complex or rare that a further opinion is necessary. Fund-holding GPs have the freedom within their limited financial resources to arrange such second opinions. Non-fund-holding GPs may well have to make an extracontractual referral to a specialist unit outside their own health authority, and such referrals are at the discretion of the purchasing authority. Even though the GP and patient may think such a further opinion desirable, it can be refused by the purchasing authority. Expectations raised in the Patient's Charter may not, after all, be met.

- How valid is it to establish rights that raise hopes, only to find that they are not effective?
- Does such a move eventually lead to better care or just to a more complaining public?

5. To be given a clear explanation of any treatment proposed, including any risks and any alternatives, before you decide whether you will agree to the treatment

Before intervening therapeutically, all professionals need informed consent from their patients. It is relatively easy to get informed and written consent before a planned procedure such as an operation. The surgeon or a member of his or her team can discuss the different techniques to be used and the chances of success and would probably briefly allude to the remote surgical, medical and anaesthetic hazards. The risk of damage to the spinal cord during surgery on the vertebral column should always be discussed, but if this is not done sensitively, nervous patients who would benefit from the surgery may be dissuaded from a procedure because of this small risk. Doctors and nurses should use their professional skills and experience to tailor their explanation to the patient and circumstances surrounding the procedure involved. For example, there is a remote risk of perforating the oesophagus and other structures when passing a nasogastric tube. If that tube is passed sensitively and carefully, the risk is extremely low. Should nurses discuss this risk before undertaking what is an uncomfortable procedure? By doing so, they may increase the apprehensiveness of their patient, the difficulty of the procedure and, therefore, the resulting risk. If the passage of that nasogastric tube was essential for the preservation of the patient's well-being, the nurse may have done him or her a disservice by too graphic a discussion of the hazards involved.

Sometimes the risks of procedures have not been fully quantified. Alternative treatments may have their own risks and benefits, yet they, too, may not be quantified. Such a situation is common in combination chemotherapy for malignant disease. The only ethically correct answer is to enrol patients in carefully controlled clinical trials and to compare the outcome of different treatment protocols. Some patients are keen to accept new treatments in the hope of an increased likelihood of cure. Others are deeply suspicious at being treated as 'guinea pigs' and might refuse consent to join such trials. The doctor, then, has no choice but to select at random one treatment option, even though the benefits and risks may not be fully known.

Our professional responsibility to obtain informed consent must, therefore, on occasion be modified. Part of this informed consent entails discussing risks of and alternatives to any particular treatment. These risks and alternatives may not always be fully known, and we should be grateful that the Patient's Charter is worded 'any risks and any alternatives' rather than 'all risks and all alternatives'.

- Is this right enough? How often is information given selectively? Can patients insist on being given more information?
- Is it possible to specify the professionals' duties?
- Patients who do not agree to certain treatments are quickly labelled as 'uncooperative'. What about such situations?

6. To have access to your health records, and to know that those working for the NHS are under a legal duty to keep their contents confidential

The right of access to health records has been confirmed by legislation (Access To Health Records Act 1990). The

Charter reaffirms this basic right, but it should be remembered that it is not retrospective. Patients have no legal right to demand access to their records prior to November 1991.

The duty to keep medical and nursing records confidential is primarily a professional one. This duty may be reinforced by the contract of employment with the NHS or NHS trust. Much sensitive clinical information is handled by non-professional staff, such as medical secretaries and ward clerks. Their only obligation to confidentiality may be a contractual one. (The author is not aware of any statutory duty of non-professional staff to keep records confidential.) The courts may occasionally override the professional and contractual obligation of employees if this is in the public interest. Contrary to the views expressed in the Patient's Charter, there may be a legal duty to divulge information, when required to do so by a properly constituted court of law. Doctors and nurses should always seek the advice of their professional bodies in such situations.

The accusation of breach of confidentiality may be used to prevent health-care workers speaking out about standards of care. On occasion, it has been used to discipline workers who have spoken out. Graham Pink, a charge nurse at Stepping Hill Hospital, Stockport, was concerned about staffing arrangements and standards of care on the wards where he worked. The patients were elderly and acutely ill and did not always have an advocate to speak on their behalf. Mr Pink's concerns did not appear to have been adequately considered by management, and he approached the press. He gave details of what he thought was unsatisfactory care without naming individual patients. The information supplied nevertheless enabled a patient to be identified, and Mr Pink was suspended and then dismissed from his post (Turner, 1992). Desmond Smith, a health visitor working with Hounslow and Spelthorne

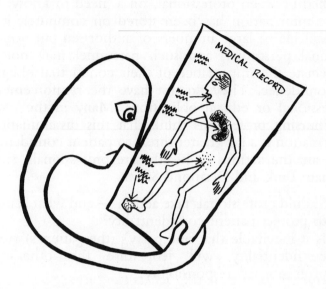

Health Authority, was also suspended and dismissed from his post. Mr Smith was concerned that a complaint against him had been racially motivated. When his employing authority failed to investigate his concern adequately, he sent clinical material in confidence to his MP. When his health authority learnt of this, he was suspended on the grounds that he had broken patient confidence. His professional body, The English National Board for Nurses, Midwives and Health Visitors, did not feel that he had any case to answer. An industrial tribunal later confirmed that view and awarded Mr Smith considerable compensation for unfair dismissal (*Health Visitors Journal*, 1993).

There are other, greater, concerns over confidentiality. Many of the changes in the health service require that large amounts of information be passed back to management, purchasing and auditing authorities. Much of this infor-

mation is specific to individual patients. It is no longer
handled between professionals on a 'need to know' basis.
Once information has been stored on computer, it may
be available to large numbers of authorised but non-professional personnel, and such personnel may not fully
appreciate the importance of their contractual obligation
of confidence. They do not have the reinforcement of
professional or ethical obligations. Many in the medical
and nursing professions think that this dissemination of
information is a far greater threat to patient confidentiality
than are the actions of health-care professionals, such as
Graham Pink and Desmond Smith.

• Should professionals take action — and what action —
  to protect patient confidentiality?
• Is it inevitable that one party's (the patient's) right to
  confidentiality will jeopardise the other's (the
  professional's) responsibility?

7. To choose whether or not you wish to take part in medical research or medical student training

It is common courtesy to approach patients for permission
to take part in research or training. New treatments are
often introduced as research protocols. Patients wishing to
benefit from advances in treatment should be encouraged
to take part in such studies. If large numbers decline,
advances in medicine will be slower and more uncertain.

Medical and nursing students require clinical experience. Attachment to clinical 'firms' in teaching hospitals is
a necessary part of building experience. Teaching hospitals
rely on this pool of student labour, and many patients
appreciate that the expertise of a teaching hospital out-
weighs any disadvantages from this. Medical and nursing
students (and those who are qualified but remain within
training grades) should always be supervised by more

senior colleagues. This supervision should be the primary safeguard for patients. If too many exercise their right to withdraw from training programmes, the experience of trainees and future standards of care may suffer, and we should make this clear to our patients.

- Is this right only partly given?
- Is it possible that patients who invoke this right might be discriminated against? How could this be avoided?

The New Patient's Charter Rights

1. To be given detailed information on local health services, including quality standards and maximum waiting times

This is the first of the three new rights introduced from 1 April 1992. Statistics for waiting times for hospital clinics and hospital admissions have been collected, collated and distributed to GPs and Community Health Councils (CHCs). In June 1994, this information was also circulated to the national press, in the form of 'league tables' of hospitals and other provider units.

There is, however, a danger of confusion in the minds of the general public over different standards and measures of quality. It is easy to measure waiting times. They may range from the number of rings before a phone is answered to the number of weeks between a GP writing to a consultant and the latter seeing an individual patient. It is much more difficult to gauge the quality of advice given when the telephone is picked up or when the specialist is seen. The outcome of an individual consultation is both confidential and affected by a multitude of factors. It has been said that the only truly reliable and measurable standard of health care is the mortality rate, but even this is open to misinterpretation. For example, one surgeon may be reluctant to risk any intervention in those who are elderly or have a particular form of disease, as he or she may genuinely feel that the risk to the patient will outweigh any benefit. A neighbouring surgeon whose skills and experience are equivalent may, however, have a more liberal attitude. Local GPs, and possibly even their patients, will be aware of this. High-risk patients who are, nevertheless, keen on intervention will be referred to the second surgeon, whose mortality figures will be higher even though this surgeon is as skilled as any colleague.

Other factors may also affect outcome. Patients with lymphoblastic leukaemia will normally receive combination chemotherapy. A high proportion of them go into a successful remission, but a few relapse. Recurrent disease may be treated by very high-dose chemotherapy and autologous bone marrow transplanation (ABMT). ABMT is very demanding of resources, and only a few regional units are able to offer this service. The complication and death rates remain high, but the alternative would be to offer relapsed patients only palliative treatment. A statistical analysis of individual treatment episodes will show that a high proportion of patients are cured at the smaller peripheral units offering standard chemotherapy. Patients who fail initial treatment or who relapse later will be referred to regional units offering ABMT. Their success rate will be lower and mortality higher, but the statistics provided must be interpreted with great caution. Statistics concerned with lesser outcomes than life and death are equally difficult to formulate and interpret.

- There is a real danger that the general public may come to equate measurable but largely irrelevant statistics such as waiting times with the relatively unquantifiable, but much more important, standard of quality of care. Should this be encouraged through the Charter?

Past experience has shown that the most popular of units with the most skilled staff have often had the longest waiting times. In essence, a form of 'rationing' by waiting had been introduced. The new reforms of the health service with 'money following patients' were intended to rectify this situation. It remains to be seen whether or not purchasers will be able to measure the true quality of provision and thus reward provider units financially, in order that they can increase their services. There is a danger that units or NHS trusts may divert resources into areas in which they know they can achieve measurable quality standards, for example routine orthopaedic surgery, and away from areas in which outcome is much more difficult to quantify, such as the provision of long-term care for those with severe learning disability and multiple handicap. It remains important that patients and their advocates have access to detailed information on health services, so that they can make an informed choice on the use of those services. That information must be prepared with scrupulous care and must be free of any political or professional bias.

• What are 'rights' given by Charter if they may not be effectively usable as rights?

2. To be guaranteed admission for treatment by a specific date no later than 2 years from the date when your consultant places you on a waiting list

The scandal of long waiting lists has been with the health service for many years. In some specialties, the waiting list has been used as a rationing device. Patients who are old or physically frail might be unable to benefit from the procedure when it is finally offered; perhaps such patients should not have been put on a waiting list in the first place. There has been some concern that long waiting lists may encourage patients to turn to the private sector. In some areas, the longest waiting lists, for example for orthopaedic surgery and ear, nose and throat surgery, correlate with the amount of private practice in those specialties in the same area. Accusations have been made that unscrupulous specialists might wish to 'line their own pockets' by not tackling their long NHS waiting lists, but instead, treating private patients. The question of whether long waiting lists encourage private practice or whether private practice is a necessary result of long waiting lists is as difficult to answer as it is to decide whether the proverbial chicken or egg comes first. Whatever the underlying reasons for these long waiting lists, the government has introduced various commendable schemes in order to reduce them. Employment of additional consultants, diversion of patients to areas with spare capacity and, most contentiously, NHS funding of private care have all been tried.

Consultants have been asked to modify their practices in order to remove patients who have been waiting for 2 years or longer from their lists. Patients may be written to and invited to reattend for assessment. Their condition may have improved or their general health may have deteriorated. In either case, they do not need to remain listed for surgery. Those who do require surgery, and have been on the list for 2 years, have their admission expedited in order to clear the backlog. This is laudable, but it does mean that other patients may be disadvantaged.

Surgeons have a professional duty to use their skills and resources to the benefit of all those in their care. This means that more urgent cases must get preference. The introduction of an arbitrary 2-year maximum waiting list period, however, means that this clinical preference may be overruled by the political imperative to clear less urgent cases.

- Ethics is about what is right and wrong, good and bad. Are such practices right? If not, why not?

3. To have any complaint about NHS services — whoever provides them — investigated and to receive a full and prompt written reply from the Chief Executive or General Manager

The NHS is a virtual monopoly. Patients who are dissatisfied with the service cannot easily take their custom elsewhere. There is, therefore, little or no commercial pressure on providers of health care to raise standards. The British people have, by and large, been very happy with the standard of care provided, but it is not easy to define satisfactory provision of services when there are no alternatives to judge them by. Complaints or criticisms of service are, however, a necessary spur to improvement, and the government is encouraging a shift from subservient patient to critical consumer.

Patients need to know to whom they should complain. A complaint may be made to a purchasing authority. These are being formed by the merger of the District Health Authorities (DHAs), which purchase community and hospital services, and FHSAs, which purchase general medical, dental, ophthalmic and pharmaceutical services. A complaint could also be made to the provider, i.e. the hospital trust, family doctor, or fund-holding practice, or to the professional bodies of the medical and nursing professions, the General Medical Council (GMC) and the United Kingdom Central Council for Nursing, Midwifery and Health Visiting (UKCC) respectively.

There is already plenty of evidence that the number of complaints has increased. The main effect of this appears not to be an improvement in standards of care but a deterioration in professional autonomy and morale. Complaints against hospital doctors are handled by the unit or

NHS trust for whom they work. Any apology or settle-
ment for damages is made by that trust. In theory, hospital
doctors no longer need to belong to a professional defence
body, although many have chosen to remain members.
They are concerned that a trust could take the easiest and
least costly course of action and admit liability, without
holding a full enquiry or defending the case within the
courts. The resultant damage to a doctor's professional
standing and job prospects could be immense.

Family doctors have also seen a surge in complaints
following the introduction of the NHS reforms and the
publication of the Patient's Charter. GPs are in triple jeop-
ardy. Firstly, complaints may be made to the FHSA that
they have been in breach of contract. At a Service committee hearing, they may be found guilty of failure to visit or
render appropriate treatment, be admonished and have
part of their remuneration withheld. Secondly, a successful
outcome at a Service committee hearing may encourage
the patient or relative with a complaint to proceed
through the civil courts with a claim for damages. Thirdly,
a complaint may also be made to the GMC, which can
discipline a doctor or remove his or her name from the
medical register, thus depriving him or her of a livelihood.

By raising expectations, the Patient's Charter encourages
complaints when those expectations are not met. Even if
complaints are directed against the health service authority
purchasing or providing care, the result is often that individual doctors become the subject of an enquiry and disciplinary action. If there has been serious malpractice or
negligence, this is appropriate. Frequently, it is lack of
training, time or resources that leads to a situation causing
a complaint to be made. Provision of these commodities
is the responsibility of the employing authority, and it is
unjust that individual doctors (or nurses) should be held
to account for any deficiency. It is clearly unethical to
raise expectations when there are insufficient resources

to meet those expectations. All professionals have a duty to highlight such discrepancies before damage is caused to patients under their care, but this course of action may be fraught with difficulty and danger. Concerns must always be expressed through the normal channels of the unit in which the professional works. Failure to do this will also invite disciplinary action. The response from the employing authority may not, however, be adequate; what is a doctor (or nurse) to do in this situation? This was the dilemma faced by Graham Pink in 1989. He could have soldiered on, done his best and in the 1990s been subject to a complaint by a patient or relative. He chose to anticipate such events, spoke out and was suspended.

The Patient's Charter may encourage complaints from patients (or their families) with personality disorders or paranoid illness or those who are constitutionally vexatious. It may be difficult for the chief executive or administrative staff of an NHS trust to interpret and evaluate these complaints. A recent example concerned the word 'degenerative' used in a letter to describe the serious inherited condition of a patient. This word appears to have been misinterpreted as 'degenerate' by the patient's mother and the administrative staff of the trust to whom the complaint was made. This misconception should be easily resolved, but formal investigation into such a complaint could reinforce the grievance felt by the mother and the distress felt by the doctor concerned.

- This right could be interpreted as a licence to complain. Should change only be made after a complaint, or should there be another 'charter' for whistleblowers? Has one party more rights than the other?

The National Charter Standards

1. Respect for privacy, dignity and religious and cultural beliefs

This is the first of the national Charter standards, as distinct from Charter rights. There has been concern that the health reforms might decrease the autonomy of the individual and the accountability of those who provide health care. Members of health authorities (the purchasers) and NHS trusts (the providers) are nominated by the Secretary of State for Health or Regional Health Authority (RHA), rather than being elected by the local population. Individual and small group practices are being replaced by larger fund-holding practices or non-fund-holding GP consortia. Health care is now being provided from larger and more remote units, and it is necessary to restate that the wishes and beliefs of individuals will be respected. There are considerable ethical and financial implications. For example, there is an increased risk of mortality in a Jehovah's Witness refusing transfusion after a road traffic accident. The length of hospital stay and cost of treatment might also be considerably higher (Finfer et al, 1994). It is essential that the necessary funding is made available to meet this standard.

Privacy and dignity are not easy to maintain on open 'Nightingale' wards and the change to smaller wards and single-bedded rooms is welcomed by many. Some units have reintroduced the concept of payment for 'amenity' beds in single rooms. We should be careful to ensure that all those who would benefit from or wish for the privacy of a single room have this opportunity, regardless of their ability to pay.

- It seems difficult nowadays not to be influenced by economy when considering ethical problems. Are economy and ethics exclusive of each other?

2. Arrangements to ensure everyone, including people with special needs, can use services

This is a laudable standard but could be open to misinterpretation. Provision of wide doors, ramps and disabled toilet facilities will ensure that many people with disabilities can use health service premises. However, accessing services will still be difficult for some, and it is necessary that doctors, nurses and others who work within the service are willing to adapt their method of working, as well as their place of work, to meet the needs of the disabled. Nevertheless, there should be a limit to the idea of 'normalisation'. Many people with disabilities will still require to be visited in their own homes in order to benefit from services. Community care teams employed by both health and social services are in an ideal position to meet the requirements of those with special needs.

• How could this standard be misinterpreted? To what extent do doctors and nurses have a duty to implement this standard?

3. Information to relatives and friends

It is not easy to pass information over the telephone to the many enquirers who phone a hospital ward each day. The bland statements 'satisfactory' or 'she had a comfortable night' are virtually meaningless, but more specific information about patients and the progress of their treatment is difficult to give confidentially. Ideally, the identity of each caller should be checked and the consent of the patient obtained before information is passed on. Such an ideal is virtually impractical on a busy medical or surgical ward.

• This is another area in which rights and responsibilities

may conflict. What could be an ethical way of solving a conflict in the area of information-giving?

4. Waiting time for an ambulance service

This Charter standard states that an emergency ambulance should arrive within 14 minutes in an urban area or 19 minutes in a rural area. There is no interpretation of the word 'should'. At present, the Department of Health regards an ambulance service as satisfactory if 95 per cent of response times lie within the stated Charter limits. Such rigid interpretation allows little leeway for individual ambulance controllers, who need to be able to use their professional discretion. Many of them are very experienced and can assess priorities over the telephone. They have an obligation to respond to all emergency calls, but they should have the discretion to prioritise these calls. They may need to divert an ambulance from a less urgent call to one they know needs an immediate response, even if this means that the first caller is waiting greatly in excess of the Charter time. If they can justify this decision, no action should be taken against them. Nevertheless, there is subtle pressure to conform to the Charter standards, and this pressure might override their own professional judgement, with disastrous consequences for the individual.

Another concern here is the accountability of ambulance services, particularly those operating as trusts. As a GP, I once had to ask for urgent assistance for a patient with a pneumothorax who lived in a very isolated cottage down a rough track. Access to the house could only be gained by four-wheel drive vehicles. The patient was very short of breath, and I arranged to stay with him until the ambulance arrived.

On telephoning the service and specifically asking for the four-wheel drive ambulance, I was told that it had been taken out of service. I expressed my surprise but settled for an ordinary ambulance and, with some difficulty, transported the patient in my own four-wheel drive vehicle to an access point that the ambulance could reach. Next morning, I discussed the problem with the director of ambulance services. He did not feel the need to justify the withdrawal of the four-wheel drive ambulance, nor did he seek to justify his omission to tell local GPs. He even expressed surprise that a local GP acting as an advocate on behalf of the consumer expected to have been told. I would prefer ambulance services to be answerable to local needs, local opinions and local democracy rather than centrally imposed, and possibly locally irrelevant, Charter standards.

- The Patient's Charter is detailing patients' rights, and professionals have their codes of ethics or practice. Should they be made to coincide? Can every area of accountability be clearly set out?
- Why does the manager's accountability seem less urgent than the practitioner's?
- How can the needs of the one be squared with the needs of the many?

5. Waiting time for initial assessment in Accident & Emergency departments

Accident & Emergency departments are notorious for long delays. This is probably unavoidable. Staff numbers are limited, and the management of patients with multiple injury takes a great deal of time. Several such patients may be admitted after a road traffic accident, so patients with apparently minor trauma may have to wait considerable periods while more serious cases are treated.

It is important that some assessment is made on arrival. In the past, this has probably been done by experienced receptionists, and the wording of the Charter standard does not prohibit such a scheme from continuing. Many units now employ a triage nurse to assess all patients on arrival. This has the advantage that a trained professional will have made an assessment, however brief, even though the patient may still wait several hours for definitive diagnosis and treatment.

Such brief assessments are not easy. I still have vivid memories of a young man who walked into an Accident & Emergency department many years ago. He had suffered an injury while playing football. He reported to the desk and sat down, while I and my colleagues attended to the occupants of two cars that had been in collision. When his name was finally called, we realised the young man had become unconscious. He was immediately transferred to another unit for evacuation of his extradural haematoma. The delay did not improve his prognosis. Even with a triage nurse, I suspect that the degree of urgency would not, in this case, have been correctly assessed. Even if patients are assessed appropriately on arrival in an Accident & Emergency department, they may become disgruntled at the delay before treatment is completed. If there is no increase in staffing, those who are assessed as non-urgent may have to wait even longer than previously, as more urgent cases are given their correct priority.

Expectations have increased. The incidence of complaints and litigation after treatment at accident departments is already high. The frequency of legal action may be increased rather than reduced because of the rise in expectations and the difficulties of maintaining a high-quality triage system.

• On the surface it may seem that this standard, too, is cosmetic rather than a right to be claimed. Should it, therefore, not have been made? Now that it exists, how can it be made to work to benefit all concerned?

6. Waiting time in outpatient clinics

It is both common courtesy and a proper use of resources
to book patients into clinics at times when they are
likely to be seen with the minimum delay. The practice
of block booking of six or eight patients at an identical
time has been rightly discouraged. Despite impeccable
organisation, an outpatient department will always be liable
to unexpected difficulties and delays. New patients, particularly in the broader specialties of general medicine and
general surgery, require enormous variation in the time
needed to resolve their problems. Follow-up patients may
present with new symptoms, requiring a complete reassess-
ment of their condition. Patients may arrive late, have to
be sent to other departments, such as X-ray, which may
have delays of their own, or be taken acutely ill on the
clinic premises, requiring urgent intervention by medical
and nursing staff. In some specialties, such interruptions
to the smooth flow of the clinic are everyday occurrences
and not exceptional.

Our first professional responsibility is to the individual
patient, but the requirement to conduct a smooth and
efficient outpatient service might impinge on that primary
responsibility. There could be subtle but irresistible pressures to hurry the interview and examination of a new
patient with a particularly complex or abstruse problem.
Patients attending for review and presenting new symptoms may be 'fobbed-off' with platitudes or else referred
to a colleague whose own clinic may be oversubscribed
and have a long waiting list. Radiology and pathology
investigations should never be embarked on lightly, as they
are expensive and may cause distress to patients. There is
the additional concern that patients referred for these tests
may have to be seen a second time in the clinic for their
results, thus either delaying the existing clinic or adding
to the workload of the next one. This additional pressure

might cause a clinician to decide against doing these tests, when the clinical balance would otherwise have been in their favour.

• The Charter standard states that patients 'will' be seen within 30 minutes of the specific appointment time given. If this is not realistic, given the difficulties described, can a manager be held responsible? How far does a 'duty to care' go in this instance?

7. Cancellation of operations

Surgeons in many specialties have to contend with routine, booked surgery and frequent emergency operations. On many surgical wards, the number of acute emergency admissions may regularly exceed the number of planned, non-urgent admissions. Many technological advances do not apply to emergency surgery. Patients may be elderly, very sick and require major procedures, such as bypass surgery for arterial blockage or bowel resection and enterostomy for malignant tumours or other obstructive diseases of the gut. Surgical teams may operate into the small hours to deal with a backlog of emergency surgery admitted during the day 'on take', even though a routine operating list may be booked the following morning. Tired junior staff are resilient and will cope, but the additional requirement of the Patient's Charter gives them yet another factor to contend with.

Medical and nursing staff do not cancel lists and inconvenience patients lightly. They already know that delayed surgery may re-present as an emergency, thus perpetuating a vicious cycle. There must be adequate theatre time, trained theatre staff and an adequate number of senior and junior surgeons to cope with both the routine and emergency workloads. Because the time and resources required for emergency work are unknown, it is difficult to gauge the spare capacity that might be required. This calculation is particularly difficult in smaller units or in those specialties, such as vascular surgery, that are highly specialised. It is not likely that any increase in resources will be forthcoming.

The Patient's Charter has been introduced alongside a policy of cost containment and a reduction in the number of hospital beds. Day-care units may be efficient and cost effective, but they are staffed by the same surgical teams who have to contend with emergency procedures. It might be better to use dedicated surgical personnel to staff these units, alongside what is often a dedicated nursing team. The staffing requirements of each unit would need to be increased and the opportunities for training would need to be safeguarded.

* Should this standard have been included in the Patient's Charter?

8. A named qualified nurse, midwife, or health visitor responsible for each patient

Personal responsibility may seem an old-fashioned concept and has a hallowed tradition. Florence Nightingale gave an illuminating reply when asked when a nurse's responsibility ended. It was her opinion that nurses remained responsible for their patients even when off duty and off the ward. Of course, they could not be there 24 hours a day, 7 days a week, but they had an individual and professional duty to hand over their patient's care to colleagues who were aware of, and knew how to meet, that patient's requirements. Despite the onset of a team approach, this doctrine of personal responsibility never quite died out. Family doctors have a personal responsibility to provide services for their patients 24 hours a day, 365 days a year. Although they share care with partners, deputies and locums, the ultimate

responsibility, nonetheless, lies with the doctor whose
name is on the medical card and who accepted responsibility for the patient when he or she agreed to provide a
service. Some GPs have found this responsibility too oner-
ous and have petitioned for change, but it is unlikely that
any alterations to this personal contract will be made.

In Florence Nightingale's day, the ward sister or senior
nurse would hold ultimate responsibility for all those under
her care. Today, sisters or charge nurses remain ultimately
responsible for the smooth running of their ward or
department. The days of the large open wards are gone,
and it would be a practical impossibility for the senior
nurse on each ward to take the same kind of personal
responsibility envisaged by Florence Nightingale. The professional duty as head of the team persists, but individual
care needs to be delegated. It is a fact of human nature
that people relate better to another individual than to a
team; a named nurse will have a relatively small number
of patients under his or her care and is in a position to act
as their advocate.

Many units have a named nurse organising outpatient
or treatment clinics, being responsible for the smooth running of the clinic. If there are delays or patients are forgotten, it may be the nurse's name that is on the clinic
notice board for everyone to see. Doctors may have some
difficulty adjusting to the idea of a named nurse. Rather
than look at the bedhead or clinic notice board to see
which nurse is responsible, they may approach the nearest
available member of the nursing staff. They can and should
be referred firmly and politely to the colleague who is
acting as named nurse.

Personal responsibility *is* compatible with professional
teamwork. It raises standards of care and restores a sense
of control to those who are receiving that care. Deficiencies in the performance of any individual nurse may be
highlighted, and it is important that these deficiencies are

corrected in a constructive and non-threatening way. It is also important that the duty rota of the named nurse is such that patients for whom she or he is responsible will see her or him reasonably frequently. This may cause practical difficulties on wards that make use of a high proportion of part-time staff (see also Chapter 1).

• This Charter standard is about organisation as well as personal responsibility. Does the fact that a nurse has a statutory responsibility lead to that nurse also being personally and professionally willing and able to carry it out?

9. Discharge of patients from hospital

This Charter standard reflects the requirements of the National Health Service and the Community Care Act 1990. Prior to a patient's discharge, an assessment of needs for community care services should be carried out. These needs might encompass the provision of community nursing services and local authority Social Services. The Charter states that the patient (and, with his or her agreement, the carers) will be consulted and informed at all stages.

The arrangements made may not necessarily satisfy the patients or their carers. For example, there has been much concern about the provision of long-stay care for the elderly and disabled. The number of NHS beds in these categories has been considerably reduced in recent years, and many people with medical or nursing needs are now looked after in nursing homes administered by private agencies or charitable trusts. Contributions, which are subject to a means test, are expected from patients or relatives towards the cost of nursing home care. The previous NHS provision had always been free at the point of delivery and was not, therefore, subject to a means test. Many elderly patients expect to pass on an inheritance to their children, and many families expect to receive such an inheritance; nursing home fees may destroy these expectations, so it is not surprising that there is resistance to the idea of long-stay care arranged in a nursing home. Families may be prepared to challenge such a decision in the courts, their case hingeing on the statutory obligation of the Secretary of State for Health to provide the requisite medical and nursing care. The promise of consultation and information in the Charter does not satisfy such families, who feel that decades of contribution to the NHS should give them greater say in the provision of long-term care without necessarily having to contribute further towards its cost.

- This last standard may, therefore, be seen to be as contentious as all the others. Will the presumed empowerment of patients and clients change the situation?
- Ethics is about what 'is' as well as what 'should be'. In the light of this, how can this standard be assured?

Conclusion

This chapter has considered the ten rights and nine standards that the Patient's Charter expects to be met or exceeded within the NHS. The Charter raises expectations and encourages complaints if those expectations are not met. It concerns itself with the more measurable aspects of health care and seeks to measure the performance of the NHS by such indices as waiting times for outpatient appointments, delays in Accident & Emergency departments and the proportion of patients treated by day surgery. This may be the Charter's undoing.

There is little attempt to measure the outcome of medical and nursing care, and quality assessments are necessarily subjective and always difficult to measure. This begs the question of whether such a Charter is helpful or should even exist.

Many people working within the NHS are concerned that extra resources are spent on administration and measurement of Charter standards, rather than on improving the quality of care. This book focuses on the ethics of the Charter and shows that these are legitimate concerns. The main purpose of the Charter is to give patients a clear idea of their rights in the health-care services they use. A list of rights will, inevitably, lead to an expectation of their fulfilment and a demand for further rights. The Charter seems to be concerned with empowering the consumer but is very vague on how expectations can be met when human and material resources are limited. At times, the Charter seems to be more concerned with image, rather than patients' rights to comprehensive and high quality health care.

Is the Charter not in danger, then, of being simply a vehicle for impressive statistics? The duty of professionals to act in their patients' best interests seems to have been subjugated to meeting the stereotyped demands of the Charter. The medical and nursing professions need to provide a service that is compassionate, responsive and of the highest quality. It is questionable that the Patient's Charter will, of itself, bring about the improvements required to meet these standards. The Charter is more likely to be seen as a stick with which the government can beat the caring professions into carrying out health policy that should more properly be under professional control. Does the Charter, then, take away from professionals their primary duty to act professionally? Does the government not trust professionals? This is one view that could be read into the Charter. Does the Charter give patients something back that was theirs by right before the government took it away by and through the market economy?

It is easier to ask questions than to give answers, and to criticise than to be constructive. The Patient's Charter seeks to answer some of the long-standing criticisms of the NHS, but it also raises many questions, some of which are of an ethical nature. Doctors and nurses have a professional obligation to make the best use of available resources and their own skills to meet their patients' needs. Who should define those needs: the patient, the professional or an elected government? However we might answer this question, the Patient's Charter is here and will not go away. Doctors and nurses should examine themselves and their professional practices in the light of its rights and standards. This may lead on to more discussion in surgeries and wards and during lectures on the Charter's implications for the ethics of health care.

References

DoH (Department of Health) (1991) *The Patient's Charter*. London: HMSO.

Finfer S et al (1994) Managing patients who refuse blood transfusions: an ethical dilemma. *British Medical Journal*, 308, pp. 1423–6.

Health Visitors Journal (1993) Health authority admits unfair dismissal. *Health Visitors Journal* 66(4), p. 114 (editorial).

Reich W (1940) The function of the orgasm. Reprinted in Rosen M and Widgery D (eds) *The Chatto Book of Dissent*. London: Chatto & Windus, pp. 359–60.

Turner T (1992) The indomitable Mr Pink. *Nursing Times*, 88(24), pp. 26–9.

CHAPTER 3

A Manager's View

Andrew Wall

The public's view is often that the managers are the only ones who have benefited from the many changes and reforms in health care; this chapter presents the managers' perspective. Managers have found themselves being squeezed from all sides in the wake of the publication of the Patient's Charter. They have new responsibilities and pressure to fulfil them, and new demands made on them that they cannot readily square with the resources given.

The manager who has written this chapter puts his views forcefully. His political opinions inform his thinking and writing about the Patient's Charter and ethics in management. This third chapter, therefore, gives a different view from the first two.

Managers might have been expected to have welcomed the Charter. It set down clear guidelines on what was expected of them. Indeed, it has been described as a tool of management. At last, managers were to have their own unambiguous role in relation to patients, no longer trailing behind their professional colleagues, seemingly at the mercy of clinical autonomy and the exclusivity that surrounds those whose main purpose is to treat and care for patients. With the publication of the Patient's Charter managers would now be able to question clinicians and to insist on adherence to preordained standards. Despite this, the response to the Charter by health service managers has been ambivalent. The reasons for their uneasiness need examining.

Managers have the prime responsibility for managing health care within the resources allocated by the govern-

ment, but they have to do this in a manner that is responsive to the needs of patients and those — the rest of the
community — who may become patients. The Patient's
Charter (1991) imposed constraints upon managers, for
example being required to work to stricter targets than
before. However, the introduction of the Charter was not
just a technical exercise; it caused other dilemmas of a
more ethical nature: for example, is it right to interfere
with medical priorities?; should the right to freedom of
choice be encouraged even when it is known that the
options are limited?; and is it right to set time standards
for ambulance services that are unrealistic in some urban
areas? How far is it reasonable for the government to
demand compliance to standards that have been devised
with little reference to those running the NHS?

The Rise of Consumerism in the NHS

The history of health care had cast patients into two classes:
those who could pay and could be dealt with as individuals,
often to the extent of remaining at home or having a
private room, and the rest of the population, who were
supplicants to clinical expertise and its embodiment, the
doctor. The 1946 National Health Service Act changed
much of that, and the founding principle, still on the lips
of politicians, was that all patients should be treated equally
according to their needs. This principle, however laudable,
did not automatically give patients rights that they could
use to their own immediate advantage. Patients were
expected to fulfil the demands of the doctor and to behave
according to the instructions of the nurse. Patient
empowerment was a long way off in the early days of the
NHS.

However, by degrees the worms began to turn, and
patients, or at least a few people, such as the Community

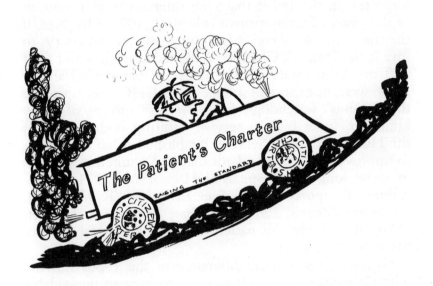

Health Councils (CHCs) (see chapter 4), founded in 1974, acting in their interests, introduced consumerist ideas onto managers' agendas. In the mid 1960s, seminal work by Professor Revans and colleagues in Manchester (Revans, 1964) established a link between patients' satisfaction with the way they were treated and the speed of their recovery. Later, Winifred Raphael and the King's Fund (Raphael, 1977) undertook surveys to find out what the patients themselves thought. Raphael included patients who might previously have been said not to know their own minds, that is, those with mental illness. Following on this came the work of Professor Brian Moores, who undertook surveys of patient opinion (Moores, 1985) that were much more searching than the five-question slip of paper that still adorns some patient lockers and is not so different from the sort of questionnaire found in hotel rooms.

These early explorers of patient opinions are too often forgotten in the belief that consumerism is an invention of the years of Conservative rule since 1979. However, if the mechanisms were there, why was it necessary to invent the Patient's Charter? Why had managers and their staff not been aware of the wishes of patients all along? They were not short of advice from CHCs, set up to be the patients' watchdogs, from pressure groups of many kinds, or, indeed, from service auditing bodies, such as the Health Advisory Service, established in an endeavour to improve the poor standards that had resulted in scandals in some long-stay hospitals (DHSS, 1969, 1971, 1978). Influential reports such as *Sans Everything* (Robb, 1967), *Put Away* (Morris, 1969) and *Home From Hospital* (Skeet, 1970) all brought the patients' experience firmly before the eyes of managers.

However, the crucial difference in the 1980s was the political climate. The welfare state, so long an unassailable edifice, was attacked by the 'new right', who were highly critical of the alleged inefficiency and unresponsiveness of the large State bureaucracies. For them, the market was an effective alternative regulated not by bureaucrats, but by users themselves: if customers are not happy with a service, they will find alternatives. Significantly, the Citizen's Charter (1991, p. 50) says:

> Whenever the client can exercise a choice, the most effective form of redress is the right of exit: the decision not to accept the service provided and to go somewhere else.

Markets are self-regulating: the inefficient die, the efficient prosper. The limitations of this ideology in a health-care setting are obvious, but some of the 'new right' ideas rubbed off on a government who were critical of the public sector, which they felt was now characterised by substantial self-interest and resistance to change. In a challenging economic climate, this was dangerous.

NHS managers were, for the most part, still locked in their belief that those who worked in the public services inhabited a higher moral plane than did managers in commerce or industry. It was, therefore, axiomatic that what they did was in the public interest and that new ideas from the commercial world were likely to be as inappropriate as they were ethically dubious. There was truth, therefore, in the view held by government that if management in the NHS would not change on its own account, it would have to be changed, either by introducing new blood or by legislation.

The first step in this revolution came with the introduction of general management in 1984, in which one person assumed overall managerial control and was accountable for the performance of the organisation. Later changes were encapsulated in the National Health Service and Community Care Act 1990 and set the NHS on a course markedly different from that arising from any of the organisational tamperings of the 1970s and 1980s. Alongside these fundamental changes was the rise, industry-wide, of an interest in quality, which had spread, at first slowly and then like wildfire, from its American protagonists in Japan in the early 1950s to become a worldwide movement by 1990.

The Conservative government linked their espousal of individual rights, epitomised by the oft-reported remark of Lady Thatcher that there is no such thing as society, with the quality movement, after the publication in July 1991 of the Citizen's Charter, subtitled 'Raising the Standard'. This document is a cunning mixture of principles with popular appeal and more slanted political ideas. While no-one is likely to challenge the importance of quality, choice, higher standards or value for money, they may be more critical of the mechanisms for achieving these. It is not necessarily the case, as stated by the Citizen's Charter (pp. 4 and 5), that the means of attaining these is only by

greater privatisation, more competition, more performance-related pay or further contracting out. Here, we see
the ethics of politics at work, whereby ideas are advanced
as though they were universal truths, whereas in fact they
are partial and ideologically loaded.

NHS managers had reason to be apprehensive when the
Patient's Charter was launched shortly after the Citizen's
Charter. The minister in charge of the Citizen's Charter,
William Waldegrave, endorsed the government's view
when, in a lecture, he later justified the new health
arrangements (Waldegrave, 1993):

> My own experience in Bristol suggests that the Chairman
> of a local Trust is now infinitely more likely to be known
> and respected locally than the mêlée of bureaucratic interests
> which he or she has replaced.

The word 'mêlée' was significant; no longer were health
service managers to hide behind the convenience of the
'hospital spokesman' appellation. Now, they were expected
to be accountable to the patients they served. Put in
this way, it was hard to take exception. However, lurking
beneath the populist appeal of putting the finger on the
accountable public servant were, and are, issues that need
exploring further.

Managers' Responses to the Patient's Charter

On the face of it, managers should have been glad to
have the Patient's Charter to enhance their increasingly
dominant position in the running of the NHS. Some
undoubtedly welcomed it with open arms. The list of
standards and the declaration of rights were a challenge,
but one that could be met. It would give managers an
opportunity not only to shine in the eyes of their
superiors — their Boards, the regions, even the Secretary

of State — but also to enhance their reputation with patients and with the public, always ready to blame all the ills of the NHS on the 'bureaucrats in grey suits'.

The quality movement had already had some influence on the NHS. A few authorities were seeking British Standard BS5750 as an assurance to customers. Most NHS Trusts and District Health Authorities (DHAs) were designating quality assurance staff. As an indication of the growing enthusiasm, new magazines devoted to the subject were published (DoH, 1994a). This awareness of the importance of quality being initially almost a separate issue now fitted well the customer orientation of the new market, which split purchasers from providers. Trusts now had the incentive to prove their excellence, as it enhanced their attraction to would-be purchasers. This was particularly marked in their dealings with GP fund-holders, who took considerable interest in the detail of the quality specification within contracts. Compliance with Patient's Charter standards was, therefore, good business for NHS Trusts.

Purchasing health authorities were also able to use the Patient's Charter as a way of demonstrating their concern for the populations they were set up to serve. A public, somewhat bemused by the organisational complexities of the new NHS, were more likely to respond positively to statements on what they were entitled to and what they could expect in service terms. The Charter, therefore, enhanced the purchaser's advocacy role, which, now that health authorities were no longer bogged down in day-to-day management issues, could be made much more of.

However, not all managers felt so positively about the Patient's Charter. Some felt that they were being made to dance to the government's tune, which of course they were. No manager could publicly reject the standards or rights proclaimed by the Charter, whatever their level of sceptism as to the ability of charters to improve matters. Such managers thought that the government was mislead-

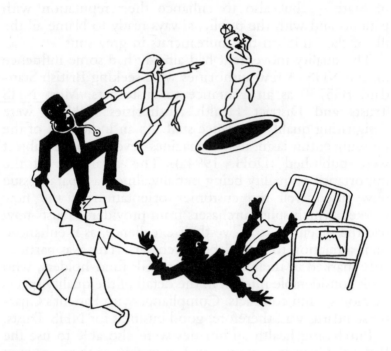

ing the public by suggesting that improving the quality of service was just a matter of trying harder, rather than providing extra resources, although some of the standards imply heavier investment in staff and supporting equipment and technology. Some managers viewed the publication of the Charter with cynicism, on the grounds that it had been designed to make the government look good, at the expense of NHS managers.

More serious was the criticism that the Charter standards would distort priorities, for example by the emphasis on shortening times spent on waiting lists. Managers found common ground with doctors in this. Doctors had been enraged that the government had intervened in the assessment of clinical priorities by dictating who should be admitted when. Not for the first, or last, time, doctors rather overreacted, but not before some managers had expressed a degree of sympathy with them.

- A fundamental ethical issue was at stake: patients should be treated according to need, rather than political opportunism.

Charter standards might have been greeted with more enthusiasm by clinicians and managers had extra resources been forthcoming. Of course, more patients could be treated, but the extra numbers would be limited without more financial investment in the NHS. The government, in its turn, had learnt to be sceptical of this way of thinking, quoting that for 10 years, they had insisted on efficiency savings, which had always been achieved, despite protests each year that it would be impossible to do so as all the fat had already been squeezed out of the system.

Managers were also concerned that the standards laid down in the Charter could be used as the basis for subsequent league tables, making invidious comparisons between one part of the NHS and another. This fear was justifiable, as regions and districts subsequently boasted about their lower waiting times, often failing to mention that they had not started from the same position and that various other factors materially affect the ability of authorities to shorten waiting times. The problem of comparisons is that, valuable though they may be as indicators for further analysis, they are also potentially dangerous if used naïvely, causing unfair and damaging opinions to be passed on to those who may be working under particular difficulties.

So what we see is the Patient's Charter being used instrumentally by government to bring about change and to call to heel the managers and the clinicians within the NHS. Those who were sceptical of the motives of the government were right to be, but, on the other hand, it was not unreasonable of the government to attempt to overcome entrenched attitudes in a public service not renowned for its ability to change practices.

This, then, was the background to the managers' response to the Patient's Charter. For those excited by the business opportunities afforded by the 1990 changes in the NHS, the Charter gave them further justification in gaining power over clinical colleagues and asserting their supremacy as the key decision-makers. The Charter also legitimised the need to limit services by being much more explicit about what could be expected — and, by implication, what could not.

Other less ambitious managers felt that their crucial relationships with clinicians could be threatened by insensitive handling of the requirements of the Charter, and they were, therefore, likely to be put in the unenviable position of trying to satisfy the government and its agents, the Management Executive and the regions, to meet the heightened expectations of patients and placate the resentment of doctors. This was not a new state of affairs, as managers have habitually been the mediators between conflicting interests, but the publicity attending the Patient's Charter made the pressure greater. In such circumstances, a code of ethics for managers might well have been welcomed, but at that time (such a code has now been proposed but not yet agreed), managers only had their own sense of what was right to guide them.

- What do we know of health service managers' approach to ethics and how does it help to analyse in more detail the implications of the Patient's Charter?

Health Service Managers and Ethics

Until recently, ethics was hardly discussed by managers. Ethics was, in their view, to do with matters of research and with large issues, such as euthanasia. The managers' role was ethically more mundane, concerned with making decisions based on the wishes of government on the one hand, and the judgements of clinicians on the other. The first book in the UK to be targeted at NHS managers and their ethics (Wall, 1989) was only published a few years ago and was greeted by many with bewilderment. Some professions were, in any case, frankly sceptical that managers' conduct was ethically based.

However, the managers' ethical agenda does not need any justification; every aspect of their work has an ethical element: as advocates of patients, as employers, as representatives of the public interest, as custodians of public funds, as upholders of the law. Their work should be informed by considerations of how best to behave. Ethics is about conduct, and managers, as 'doers', need to have a framework to help them. The problem is that there are various ways of constructing such a framework.

One approach is to concentrate on *benefits*. In this case, ethical behaviour is determined by maximising benefits. The managers' role is to ensure that the greatest number of people receive benefit from the actions of managers and other staff. This is known, broadly speaking, as utilitarianism. It is clear that the Patient's Charter responds to this idea of maximising the number of patients likely to benefit. However, this near-obsession with numbers is also a reason for criticism from clinicians and others. Quantity, in itself, is not necessarily good or, indeed, right. The concept of maximising benefit needs to elucidate the difference between how many and to what standard. In other words:

• which is more ethical, a mediocre, if adequate, service for a large number or a high-quality service for a few?

This theory of ethics begins to fall apart under this line of questioning.

An alternative view is one based on the *rights* of the

individual. Indeed, the placing of the apostrophe in 'Patient's' makes the point that the Charter is for each individual, rather than for patients in general: it is 'my charter'. Ethically, the individual rights movement has considerable power, particularly with individual empowerment now being a central doctrine of politicians of all persuasions. The difficulty that arises, however, is that one person's right may deny another's. Where there are limited resources, choices have to be made.

- Is it right to deny treatment for infertility to women on the grounds that the purchasing health authority has to ration choices in order to live within their allocation?
- How much money should be spent on the unconscious, severely injured road accident patient?
- Is it right to means test an elderly person needing social care when she or he has paid into the State through taxes and might, therefore, expect to be treated the same as any other fellow citizen?

Individual rights, which in the USA (although not in the UK) are enshrined in a constitution, are the life blood of the Charter approach, but honouring them imposes almost insurmountable problems on managers and clinicians alike.

For many clinicians, the debate may appear too convoluted. They are governed by codes of conduct that make their position clear: simply, they are to do the best for their patients. We might call this the ethics of *care*. In order to fulfil the obligations of this approach, professionals must ensure that they are properly trained in the first place and subsequently maintain their skills. Much in the Patient's Charter echoes this approach. The problem is a managerial one.

- What is to be done if the resources are insufficient to honour the wishes of clinicians?

- What if the care proposed is too expensive or the equipment not easily available?

Ethical fundamentalists refuse to be troubled by these practical details. They will say that we all have a *duty* to do what is right for our patients, and, if this is constrained, it is the responsibility of government, acting as our representative, to resolve the matter. What, after all, is the role of government if it is not to be the servant of the citizenry who elected it? This type of rhetoric may rouse the masses, but managers will find it useless in day-to-day decision-making. The Patient's Charter does not avoid rhetoric in phrases such as 'The National Health Service is the envy of the world' and 'always puts the patient first'. Sceptics might point out that if the NHS were so universally admired, the Patient's Charter would not be necessary.

One way of reducing the ethical dilemma of having to choose between one patient and another is to develop some agreement on who is the more deserving, what might be called the ethics of *virtue*. Clinicians are scandalised with this approach, as it allows judgements to be made on lifestyle rather than on clinical need. Nevertheless, it clearly tempts managers and some members of the public.

- Is it really worth rewarding patients by treating the consequences of their bad behaviour?

The smoker has, after all, been warned that he or she is increasing the risk of heart and other fatal or crippling diseases. The male homosexual indulging in plural sexual contacts increases his risk of AIDS. The obsessive overeater is more likely to have a stroke. Justification for restricting care of these patients can be made on the grounds that the outcome of treatment is likely to be less favourable, but the same can be said of the person with learning disability, the elderly confused and the baby with a congenital birth defect.

In approaching the Patient's Charter from an ethical standpoint, managers find that their position is compromised by conflicting ethical perspectives. None of the ways described above give a cast-iron approach that might give the manager an ethical template against which decisions can be made. The Patient's Charter similarly lurches from one ethical perspective to another, never resolving the fundamental dilemma of whether it is really about maximising the rights of the individual or the benefits of the population at large. This confusion is made worse by other published health policy, such as *The Health of the Nation* (DoH, 1992). However, it is not reasonable to expect a totally consistent view when philosophers over thousands of years have been unable to agree.

Purchaser and Provider Roles

At first glance, it seems that the providers of health care are more likely to be held accountable for implementing and honouring the Patient's Charter. In fact, purchasers also have an important role. Firstly, they have to help the public to know what they can expect. For the lay person, the complexity of the NHS is daunting. It is doubtful whether or not the public has a clear perception of the differences between purchasers and providers. They cannot be expected to understand concepts such as health gain without considerable explanation. And, it has to be said, they may not care. Their requirements are that when they need them, the services should be available. Ethically, this poses a problem for the health authorities.

• How far should health authorities endeavour to help the public understand the new organisation and the relative responsibilities of each part of that system?

It is fine to espouse patient empowerment, but, in so

doing, authorities cannot force patients into considering issues and facing choices if they do not wish to.

Purchasers, therefore, are most likely to be informed by their own professional judgements, initially working prospectively to ensure that the rights and standards of the Patient's Charter are incorporated into their specifications. However, there has, to date, tended to be a gap in the purchasing cycle, which has serious implications. Setting standards and stating rights does not ensure that they are observed; how are purchasing authorities to ensure that their prospective providers will comply? To check after contracts have been awarded is too late. It is here that accreditation should enter the purchasing cycle, but, to date (1994), the accreditation of intending providers is rudimentary. If purchasers are to safeguard the public, they should not be inviting tenders for provision from those whose standards are not acceptable. There is some ambivalence on the government's part here. In the early days of the changes, they were anxious that the purchaser–provider split should become a reality, and the different roles were, therefore, exaggerated to avoid collusion between managers who had previously been in the same organisation. This had the side effect that purchasers were discouraged from showing too close an interest in the way in which providers conducted themselves. Providers, jealous of their new independence, were unlikely to take kindly to enquiries about process and were only prepared to give information about outputs and, with less confidence, outcomes. There were, and indeed are, dangers in this. To assure the public, it must be necessary for the purchasers not only to set standards, but also to be knowledgeable about the quality of the process. To providers, that may look like interference.

More attention has been given to monitoring by purchasers, and extended guidance has been issued by the National Health Service Management Executive

(NHSME), not only on what to monitor, but also on
exercises in sampling techniques. Such didactic 'top-down'
advice has scarcely exemplified the ethical principle of
recognising the sovereignty of the individual. Purchasers
are in danger of being treated as process workers with no
independent ethical sense. This is dangerous because,
under such a close requirement to stick to the rules, actions
are taken not on their merit but merely to satisfy the
superior level in the hierarchy.

A somewhat critical recent examination of the Patient's
Charter (Hogg, 1994) sums up the purchaser's role in
a short paragraph on the grounds that the Charter is
fundamentally about the relationship of the individual
patient to the health service. The purchaser's role is to plug
gaps, ensure that services meet specification and ensure
that users are involved in the monitoring process. The
purchasers' ethical agenda suggests much more. They are
to scrutinise the needs of the total population and prepare
local plans to meet those needs. They then have to find
providers capable of providing services of a proper standard. Contracts have to be written covering not only what
is required, but also how and at what cost, with outcome
measures that allow the success or otherwise of the contract
to be assessed. Finally, there has to be an evaluation of
how successful the whole process has been in meeting
both the needs of the community and the requirements
of central government.

However, it is easy to see why the provider's role is
emphasised. Providers are, after all, in contact with the
patient. They are responsible for the quality of the patient's
experience. It is also easier to set up programmes for
quality control in a service in which there is a clear
relationship between the supplier and the consumer. The
results are much more likely to be measurable in an unambiguous manner. Checking the timing of clinics is simple
compared with the purchaser's obligation to inform the

public about health services. So, it is not surprising that the Charter has been accepted with more enthusiasm by managers in institutions.

The Public and the Patient's Charter

At the heart of the NHS, and probably other public services, is a deep-seated ambivalence about the public. Managers will say that they work in the public sector because they have a desire to serve the community. However, as managers, they are also satisfying another impulse, which is to make decisions and achieve results. They are 'turned on' by action, hence the success of the implementation of the 1990 changes. These two impulses are sometimes at odds and may lead to a suspicion that health service managers are not in fact very responsive to public opinion, preferring to trust their own judgement in the interests of making progress. It is here that their lack of an ethical code may be most noticeable. They may appear to use public opinion in a manipulative manner, choosing what suits them in their battles against other parts of the organisation, or setting one part of the community against another. This is not unique to the NHS and can be found equally potently in, for example, the education and transport services.

To justify managers' insularity is not difficult. They will point out that despite the political rhetoric, which depends for its legitimacy on the life blood of public opinion, there is ample evidence that the public neither knows nor, in many cases, wishes to be involved. Those managers who are not cynical will attempt to explain this by pointing out the dangers of over-explicitness. What can be provided is often defined in terms of what cannot be provided; the positive requires the negative. So, some commentators (e.g. Hunter, 1993) suggest that some sort of 'muddling through' would be better, with everyone trying to do their best, even if that leads to variations in standards. This approach has some similarities with those philosophers who have suggested that random allocation of health-care resources could be as fair as any other system, given the complexity of the arguments touched upon earlier in looking at ethical frameworks.

The trouble is that neither of these approaches is likely to gain much legitimacy with the public, now that it has been alerted to its rights by the various Charters in the public services. Many, but not all, patients or passengers previously prepared to wait and grumble will now do neither, arming themselves instead with their Charter and seeking out the nearest manager.

• It is difficult to argue against the Charter movement, because the only alternative seems to undervalue consumers, which means all of us.

The ethical consequences, when it comes to matters of choice, are even more difficult, as will be discussed later.

Purchasers have, therefore, to set about involving the public in the setting of standards and the declaration of rights. Early criticism of the Patient's Charter was that it was issued from the government with scant involvement of the general public. In consequence, it may have been seen as an exercise in public relations. As Health Rights (Hogg, 1994) has pointed out:

> The value of patients' charters lies in the process of negotiating between service providers and users . . . They can be an effective way of developing more equal relationships.

To date, the evidence is that many purchasers and providers have still to make significant progress in involving users in decisions about policies and priorities. This is scarcely surprising, given the ignorance about the organisation of the NHS and given the complexity of some of these issues. The Patient's Charter is, in any case, not a good vehicle for this more profound discussion. A survey of 2000 people undertaken by the Royal College of Nursing (RCN, 1994) found substantial ignorance among the public and went on to suggest that 'to date the Charter's benefits are more tangible for managers than for patients'. So, the communication is failing in both directions. The public does not know what is in the Charter, and the managers have not adequately established what the public thinks or the choices they would support.

However, this is to generalise. There are well publicised means of involving the public (DoH, 1994a). Market research-type surveys, questionnaires through the post, focus groups gathering together people with like needs or interests — all have been tried and reported on.

- What is missing is a trusting environment in which the relationship between service supplier and service user can flourish.

The constant media pressure on the NHS, the frustration of many people working in it, the rapid changes and the lack of confidence in the integrity of managers have all created a turbulence against which almost any attempt to create a fruitful partnership might seem doomed. Nevertheless, that is the challenge to management. It is uniquely placed to establish a trusting climate. Integrity is only obtained over time and with painstaking work with the community. Clinical and other staff serving that community also need to trust managers if they are to be good missionaries. Ethics is not a 'quick fix'.

'Will' and 'Should'

Both 'will' and 'should' are used in the Patient's Charter.

* What is the significance of this?
* Indeed, what is the difference between rights and standards?

The seven existing rights are said to be 'well established', but there is a degree of wishful thinking here. Receiving care according to clinical need, regardless of the ability to pay, is scarcely borne out by the first few years of fund-holding, during which the latent 'two-tierism' of the service has become much more visible. Not only can patients jump waiting lists when they have the money to do so, but so can their GPs if they are fund-holders. Another right is to be referred to a consultant 'acceptable to you'. This right is somewhat notional for most people, who would not know the virtues of Dr X as opposed to Dr Y. The access to medical records is a bland reassurance, which, on investigation, proves not to be so unequivocal: the doctor and the legal medical record custodian, the manager, may restrict access if it is deemed by the doctor not to be in the interests of the patient to see the full record. Of the new rights, the guarantee to be admitted within the set time limit — initially 2 years, now reduced for some conditions — has not been universally honoured.

* If the rights cannot be absolutely adhered to and supported by law, are they anything more than cosmetic?

Managers have found the statement of rights helpful because it gives a clear indication of what is expected of them, and failure to achieve it is considered to be poor performance, which may, in turn, mean that they do not receive their bonus of performance-related pay. However, for the patients themselves, the rights may not be as powerful as they appear. No-one can be taken to court; doctors and managers still have some discretion, which patients may feel is not used in their interest.

The fact that the Charter is not as powerful as it looks may not matter ethically, but there is a hint of deception in these declarations. As statements of good intent, they do not attract criticism, but as 'rights' when compared with fundamental and inviolable rights, they may appear rather vapid.

If the imperative 'will' proves to be less obligatory than it appears, do the standards suffer in the same way? The problem is that, with the best of intentions, managers cannot always ensure their observance. Take, for instance, 'Practical arrangements should include meals to suit all dietary requirements' and 'private rooms [should be available] for confidential discussions with relatives'. In both cases, it is sometimes impractical to provide anything but a token special diet, particularly one that requires elaborate religious observance in its preparation. Neither, in a busy ward with six-bedded bays, can all discussions be in private. Adapting hospitals for disabled people is not a new standard; it was embodied in the Chronically Sick and Disabled Persons Act as long ago as 1970 and yet is still not fully complied with, owing to the costs of building adaptation.

The more, therefore, that the rights and standards are examined, the more they appear to be good intentions rather than anything else. That is not to say that they are not valuable, and there is a determination to hold the managers accountable through the Chief Executive to the NHS Executive. The only ethical issues are, firstly, whether users are being misled and, secondly, the dubious way in which managers are being forced to comply, by having their income threatened.

- Should high-mindedness on behalf of patients be used to coerce managers in a punitive manner?

Such paradoxical behaviour is scarcely likely to get the best out of them.

Information for Patients

Fundamental to the Patient's Charter is freedom of information. The first sort of information is about services. There should be no difficulty in providing a clear schedule of these. Managers need to decide how this can best be done. There may, however, be ethical problems with giving details of what services are not to be provided. Managers may be tempted not to mention exclusions, on the grounds that few people will notice. Once it is stated that a service is not to be contracted for, protest is likely to arise. Here again, we see the pitfalls that arise from explicitness. But there can be little argument that people have a right to know what is not being provided, as much as what is.

More difficult is the provision of information to individual patients and their relatives and carers. There is a mismatch between what doctors say patients can tolerate and what patients themselves want to know. Doctors may insist that bad news is bad for morale, and it is for the doctor to decide, as part of his or her ethic, what is in the best interests of the patient. Do managers have any say in what is good or bad for morale? Often not, because they will have no access to these dilemmas, which take place in the clinic or at the bedside. However, managers have a wider responsibility for ensuring that the issue of bad news is discussed at some point and that there is some protocol that helps all members of the therapeutic team, not only doctors. After the doctor has gone, the patient may well turn to the nurse and ask her or him what is going to happen. The nurse needs to know how to reply; the manager needs to ensure that she or he knows.

The publication of information regarding performance is very much the responsibility of the manager; this has caused some difficulty. Is it reasonable to publish each named consultant's waiting times for being seen or the length of the waiting list? On the face of it, this is information that should be shared, but doctors have put another point of view which cannot be totally disregarded. Inferences may be made about doctors with short waiting times and lists, i.e. that they have a poor reputation with GPs and, therefore, have a low level of referrals. On the other hand, the consultant may be very conscientious and keep his lists low. The problem is that the public do not know which interpretation is right, and there is no way in which the manager can influence the situation. Equally, it is a well-established accusation that some consultants keep their waiting times and lists long in order to stimulate private practice.

Should managers be part of this and similar conspiracies? Obviously not, but again there is little that a manager can do. On balance, the patient has a right to this information, but the position is ethically not as clear cut as managers would like. Similarly, any other information on performance may be subject to several interpretations, which may need further explanation by managers if unjust imputations are to be avoided.

* Who should check performance?

This is done at various levels. Firstly, the non-executive directors of the DHAs and NHS Trusts need to be able to monitor the performance of their own organisations. This requires expertise and, therefore, training. At the next level, there are those acting as the public's advocates, such as CHCs, pressure groups and local authorities. They are likely to be able to bring more knowledge than can the person in the street to the interpretation of what they are told. This, however, does not remove an obligation for health authorities and Trusts to find ways of explaining to the lay person what is happening. There is, however, a danger that such explanations dwindle into gross oversimplification and, with their language of public relations, are greeted with suspicion rather than welcomed. Managers have a particular responsibility here.

Information is also to be supplied on other quality measures. It is for management to decide how many of these should be publicised. There may be a diminishing benefit from overdoing the communication. For example, standards of communication between hospital and GP are undoubtedly a quality measure worth stating in contracts and have obvious benefit for the patient's fluent treatment, but it may not be necessary to let the public know that compliance with this standard is part of the contract.

- Communication is not about telling everyone everything; it requires more discrimination if those messages that are really important are to be received and understood.

Access

The fundamental principle of the NHS is for patients to receive health care on the basis of need, regardless of the ability to pay.

- How is this principle observed, faced with the increasing pressure on resources and the apparent need to ration access?

It has to be said that the Charter does little to resolve the dilemma of who shall have what. In the discussion above of the various ethical frameworks, it was established that no one ethical stance met all circumstances, so that maximising benefit was sometimes in direct opposition to maximising individual rights. The Charter has nothing to say on this problem; indeed, how could it? However, the rhetoric surrounding it suggests that, in some way, the Charter provides a guarantee for treatment. The key words in the first right are 'on the basis of clinical need'. This is a minefield that managers cannot avoid merely because they are not clinicians.

The assessment of need is often presented as a pseudo-science, with inputs, process and outcomes. In fact, it is value-laden and political. An ethics exercise undertaken by the author in classes with professionals of many health service groups, clinical and otherwise, has asked them to rank patients for urgency of treatment. The list of patients includes young and old, men and women, homosexuals and heterosexuals, working and the unemployed, those with chronic conditions and those who will recover as a result of treatment. The great majority of participants came to the same conclusion: the most deserving of treatment is a man with children who, after his treatment, will be able to return to work. In justifying this conclusion, socio-economic factors predominate over clinical ones. What is learnt is that establishing need is by no means easy but that consensus, even among clinical staff, may be achieved on non-clinical criteria. So what is the manager's role in this? Before it is decided not to purchase or provide certain services, there ought to be a discussion of the ethical issues involved. It has already been shown that treatments for certain conditions, such as infertility, are not considered worthy of purchase by many health authorities under the NHS. However, what has been missing is a well-conducted ethical debate before the decision has been made.

• If the implications of the Charter were to be taken more seriously, would such debates be standard practice?

The NHS reforms themselves have introduced a further

dilemma concerning access, that of GP fund-holding. Again, this is an example of one ethical stance fighting another. If we respect the rights of the individual, the advocacy of the GP on our behalf at a given moment in time is right. However, if we believe that the NHS should endeavour to treat all people equally, the effects of GP fund-holding are wrong, in that they improve some people's access to care at the expense of others'. Politicians and some GPs argue that this is not so but that improving one person's position does not correspondingly disadvantage another's. This is unlikely to be the case where resources are limited and the whole is fixed, only the size of the parts being discretionary.

- Does the market system improve or worsen patient access?

For those patients who are mobile and articulate, the new arrangements are probably an improvement, as they can put pressure on their GPs, fund-holding or otherwise, to improve access to treatment. However, for others, unable to travel significant distances because of transport problems or dependants, the situation may be worse and the Charter's assurances of little value. There is a further potential risk arising from the Charter's assurances, that patients who cannot be treated easily in the NHS may put pressure on their GPs or their purchasers to obtain treatment from the private sector. There is no bar to doing this, but the consequences may be to corrupt the system. Consultants, knowing that they can benefit from such an arrangement, may do little to improve access for NHS patients. Trust providers have limited power to interfere with what one of their consultants does in his or her own time, even if it is to enter into a separate contract with an NHS purchaser.

Choice

The freedom to choose is one of the cardinal beliefs of the market system, because the market works through choice. Those who get chosen succeed, those who do not, fail. This is consumer power at its most bald, with the right to exit the system its greatest weapon. However, the NHS cannot operate on these lines. Firstly, exiting the system by some makes the costs to those who remain greater. This is already being demonstrated in the education system, in which some schools get worse as parents who are able to do so remove their children. If a similar situation arose in the NHS, some district general hospitals would have to remain open, although at high cost and with increasing problems in maintaining clinical standards.

Secondly, if access is to be available to all, this requires a reasonable distribution of services, whatever their levels of market efficiency or geographical disposition.

Thirdly, the public may not always make the right choice. It is doubtful that the same priority would be given to the care of mentally ill people by a referendum as is given by purchasing health authorities. Nevertheless, patients can be helped to improve their own choices through the requirements of the Charter to give clear explanations of the nature of the proposed treatment and its likely outcomes. More could be done by managers to stimulate patient learning generally, using educative principles to supplement explanations by clinical staff. Diabetic centres are already establishing the benefits to patients of systematic learning, enhancing patients' ability to share in the management of their own condition.

However, the prime difficulty, in Charter terms, with the concept of choice is that, within a fixed level of resources, choice is limited. It is, firstly, limited by the ethic of fairness: it is unfair for some people to have more

than they need, even if that is their choice. Secondly, it is
unfair to have something for which there is only a marginal
need. Thirdly, it is ethically wrong that by their choice,
people deny someone else. To be fair to the Patient's
Charter, it does not go as far as offering patients unlimited
choice; in fact, it offers them very little other than to
choose a GP and to ask for a second opinion. The rhetoric
of choice has been attached to the NHS not so much
through the actual conditions of the Charter as by the
commentary by politicians and supporters of the NHS
changes anxious to demonstrate that the new NHS is more
responsive than the old. Certainly, the Charter is dedicated
to responsiveness through its various conditions, covering
more explanations, better complaints systems and the concept of the named nurse. Overall, however, the concept
of choice is dangerous for managers, who are likely to be
more attracted to utilitarian ethics, based on the maximising of benefits to the greatest number.

Respect for the Individual

Nevertheless, this is not to say that managers would wil-
lingly return to the open wards, the long queues for want
of appointment systems and the generally low priority
given to patients' personal needs. It is possible both to
maximise benefit and to be sensitive to the individual —
up to a point. It is noticeable that single rooms, personal
telephones and well-spaced appointment times, as much
as the more significant benefits of ensuring the doctor of
one's choice and the time of admission, are what often
attract patients to the private sector. Clearly there are
environmental improvements to be made within the NHS,
and the Charter requires these.

However, a quiet and sympathetic environment is easier
to achieve than the respect for confidentiality where ethical

choices have to be made on what really is in the patient's best interest. It is customary for clinicians to maintain that confidentiality is an absolute principle that they would be unwilling to transgress. Nevertheless, there are situations in which it is not immediately clear as to what is the right thing to do. For example, in a child protection case, who should be present at the case conference? Most professional staff would reserve attendance to themselves, but what if a significant witness is a volunteer play leader from the child's primary school who was the first to report the abuse and in whom the child has often confided?

- Can a non-professional be trusted to observe the rule of confidentiality, or must the case conference rely on a second-hand account related through another professional?

The problems of confidentiality usually emerge for managers from enquiries by the police and from the media. They may have to make a judgement between the rights of the individual patient and the duty to society. Indeed, managers are better placed than clinicians to make such judgements. The clinician has a professional contract with his or her patient. The manager has a general, rather than a particular, duty to the patient, to which must be added a regard for the public interest.

Professional Standards

The Charter honours the skill and dedication of the professional staff in the NHS, but managers also have a duty, with their professional colleagues, to demonstrate this.

- How can managers demonstrate their duties?

The new purchasers have been slow to explore accreditation systems, which would assure the public that only those providers who were capable would be employed to satisfy health contracts. It is assumed, perhaps too readily, that all staff are appropriately trained and equipped to undertake their role. The evidence is more disturbing. The Confidential Enquiry in Peri-Operative Deaths reports have demonstrated that surgical outcomes vary beyond acceptable limits and that some hospitals have surgeons and anaesthetists who have poor results when assessed against their colleagues elsewhere (Royal College of Surgeons, 1989 onwards). Fund-holders have been quicker than health authorities to change their referral patterns when they are dissatisfied with clinical standards. Managers in purchasing organisations need also to ensure the quality of professional practice in other groups. This requires access to clinical situations and clinical records. Audit needs to extend across the clinical team and not only be reserved for the closed world of specialty meetings. The Patient's Charter is meaningless unless the prime purpose of the NHS, the proper treatment and care of patients, is assured. Contract specifications need, therefore, to contain more requirements to demonstrate good process, good practice and good outcomes than they generally do at present.

Continuity of Care

A common complaint from patients concerns discharge arrangements. This has long been the case, and the problem has been accelerated by the increasingly shorter lengths of stay, the reduction in numbers of longer-stay beds and financial pressures on Social Services departments. The Charter endeavours to overcome these difficulties by stating that hospitals will make appropriate arrangements before discharge—but this is easier said than done. The reorganised NHS has imposed barriers that interrupt the continuum of care. No longer is the transfer of a patient from one hospital to another necessarily a simple matter as it may now involve a transaction across a Trust boundary. Furthermore, Trusts have reasons to keep patients who are financially advantageous to them and to get rid of those who are not. Social Services departments are now required to assess the means of clients and also to place the large majority of those who need residential care in the independent sector. Here, we see government policies at odds with each other, which no amount of assurances in the Charter can resolve.

Complaints

Just as discharge arrangements have been a source of continual dissatisfaction, so has the way in which complaints have been handled in the NHS. It is vain to point out that the number of complaints is infinitesimal, compared with the number of patient contacts; the quality of the service is often judged not by what went well but by what went wrong. Despite the detailed recommendations of the Davies Committee in 1974, (DHSS and the Welsh Office, 1974), and numerous ministerial statements since, the small but significant number of patients who complain have often felt the procedure to be loaded against them. Because of this, the Charter tries to pin responsibility down, naming the chief executive as the correspondent and the person to whom complaints should be addressed. This attempt to force the accountability issue is understandable, and managers have taken it to heart, but it has to be said that there are circumstances in which the patient's interest might be better served by an answer coming from a doctor or another clinician. Managers are seldom convincing in matters of clinical detail and may be positively misleading. This Charter right has now been followed up by the recommendations of the Wilson Committee (DoH, 1994b).

Is the Charter Better for Patients?

*   Is the Charter likely to improve services to patients?

The case against charters is strong. Firstly, there is the confusion between being a consumer and being a citizen; they are not synonymous. Many citizens are not consumers, and, in any case, the idea of consumerism is centred around taking, rather than contributing. Citizens enter into a mutual contract with other citizens to improve the quality of society; consumers buy, or do not buy, according to wish and take no responsibility for the production difficulties of the producer. In NHS terms, this means that managers are seen as separate from the average citizen and are judged only on whether they have succeeded or failed in producing a better NHS. This might be fair had managers unlimited resources. In fact, they have to administer what society has, through the ballot box, decided to spend on health services. That this may not be seen as sufficient is not their fault. Confusing citizen status with being a consumer weakens the idea of corporate responsibility, which many would maintain is the basis of our society.

Why then has government invested so heavily in the idea of charters? Detractors would say that charters have symbolic value, representing to the electorate a caring government concerned for the welfare of the public, particularly, in this case, those who are sick. For managers in the NHS, this is uncomfortable, because it suggests an alliance of government and public against the management. The Charter, as a symbol, is there to reassure. The very use of the words 'your rights' aims to reduce anxiety and to convince an increasingly sceptical public that the NHS is 'all right after all', once a few operational difficulties have been overcome. Detractors would say that the recent reorganisation, the failure adequately to acknowledge the changes in demography and technology and the commensurate increases in State funding all lead to a conclusion that the NHS is far from being 'all right after all'.

Another criticism of the Charter is that it increases demands on the NHS without offering the means of meeting all those demands. The reduction of time on the waiting lists has been achieved only with difficulty, and overall numbers on lists have not been reduced. Patients who were once prepared to wait for their local hospital may now be encouraged to use their Charter rights to insist on treatment elsewhere, which may, as was explored above when discussing choice, be to the detriment of another patient.

• Is it ethical to excite demand if it is unlikely that it can be met?

Finally, the Charter could be criticised because it endorses a faulty idea of human motivation. At the beginning of the Citizen's Charter, it is made quite explicit that the government believes that one of the ways of improving public services is through performance-related pay. Detractors of this theory — and that is all it is, as the evidence is not necessarily convincing — say that workers, in this case NHS staff, will cooperate only with resentment, because it is assumed that they are only working for money and that their idealism and altruism are not being acknowledged (IHSM, 1991; IMS, 1993). This elicits the cynical response that culminates in satisfying the letter rather than the spirit of the Charter in order to achieve the bonus. The Patient's Charter is, therefore, just one more device for whipping managers into shape and will not lead to a fundamental change in attitudes to patients.

However, these criticisms may appear to many to be unduly harsh and pessimistic. There can be little argument that public services in this country could do with improvement, that they have, in many ways, become insensitive to the needs of their users and that there has been too complacent a belief in the supremacy of health professionals over their patients. Lack of information, impoliteness and long waiting times have been characteristics of the NHS and do not require resources to put them right. Any manager knows that patients' tolerance of poor physical conditions is high, providing they are treated kindly and with dignity. Indeed, concentrating too much on the physical environment can actually excite patients' criticisms, as they see money being spent on inessentials.

The Patient's Charter aims to be explicit so that patients know what to expect. It is entirely reasonable that they should be clear about the standards of performance laid down for the NHS. This empowers patients; they are no longer the victims of an arcane process, the detail of which is largely shielded from their view. Once they are empowered, they can enter into a partnership with NHS staff and management, allowing a complementary discussion on what is to be done and how. It is, therefore, now possible to share care with a named nurse to plan the next stage of treatment. The new climate also allows for more explicit advocacy, through the CHCs, pressure groups or personal representatives. In the new culture, such pressure is less likely to be resented by staff and will be accepted as normal.

In this way, the knowledge base is always increasing, which, in due course, may lead to a more potent involvement of all citizens in major decisions about policies, priorities and the level of funding for the NHS. This is very much in the managers' interest. At present, they are seen as wasting time and money, which, it is assumed, would be better spent on front-line staff. A more realistic view of the value of effective management in a complex organisation would lead to a more mature understanding of what the NHS can do to improve the health of the nation.

Conclusion

It is possible to argue that the Patient's Charter is just another public relations exercise by a government obsessed with reconstructing the decaying welfare state, which, in their view, no longer serves the interests of the nation. 'Charterism' is a tool to help the person in the street to rise up and take part in this revolution against the servants of the State, who, until recently, had been all too secure from the pressures facing a late 20th century Western economy. Ethics has little to do with such an interpretation, which is based on theories of power and politics.

However, for many, such a florid 'macro' view is in danger of obscuring the advantages that the Charter initiative can produce. This is not to say that such improvements in services could not have been achieved in any case or, indeed, that the quality movement in the NHS only started with the Patient's Charter, but it has provided a catalyst for focusing on improvement and re-evaluating the relationship between users and services. The Charter can provide a check, a balance, a stimulus and a reminder that, ethically, the NHS stands as being a brave attempt to maximise the benefits to the whole of society, while honouring obligations to each particular patient. Managers have their place in endeavouring to resolve this seeming paradox.

References

DHSS (1969) *Report of the Committee of Enquiry into Allegations of Ill-Treatment of Patients and other Irregularities at Ely Hospital* (Howe Report), Cmnd 3795. London: HMSO.

DHSS (1971) *Report of the Farleigh Hospital Committee of Inquiry,* Cmnd 4557. London: HMSO.

DHSS (1978) *Report of the Inquiry into Normansfield Hospital,* Cmnd 7357. London: HMSO.

DHSS and the Welsh Office (1974) *Report of the Committee of Enquiry into Hospital Procedure* (Davies Report). London: HMSO.

DoH (Department of Health) (1991) *The Patient's Charter.* London: HMSO.

DoH (Department of Health) (1992) *The Health of the Nation,* Cmnd 1986. London: HMSO.

DoH (Department of Health) (1994a) *Involving Local People.* Leeds: NHS Executive.

DoH (Department of Health) (1994b) *Being Heard: The Report of a Review Committee on NHS Complaints Procedures* (Wilson Report). Leeds: NHS Executive.

HM Government (1991) *The Citizen's Charter.* London: HMSO.

Hogg C (1994) *Beyond the Patient's Charter: Working with Users.* London: Health Rights.

Hunter D (1993) *Rationing Dilemmas in Health Care.* Research Paper no. 8. Birmingham: NAHAT.

IHSM (Institute of Health Service Management) (1991) *Individual Performance Review in the NHS.* London: IHSM.

IMS (Institute of Manpower Services) (1993) *Pay and Performance: the Employee Experience.* London: IMS.

Moores B (1985) From the patient's mouth. *Health and Social Service Journal,* 22 August, pp. 1040–2.

Morris P (1969) *Put Away.* London: Routledge & Kegan Paul.

Raphael W (1977) *Patients and their Hospitals.* London: King's Fund.

Revans R W (1964) *Standards for Morale — Cause and Effect in Hospitals.* London: Nuffield Provincial Hospitals Trust.

Robb B (ed.) (1967) *Sans Everything — A Case to Answer.* London: Nelson.

RCN (Royal College of Nursing) (1994) *Unchartered Territory: Public Awareness of the Patient's Charter,* Report no. 000401. London: RCN.

Royal College of Surgeons (1989 onwards) *Confidential Enquiry into Peri-Operative Deaths.* London: RCS.

Skeet M (1970) *Home from Hospital.* The Dan Mason Nursing Research Committee. London: Macmillan.

Waldegrave W (1993) *The Reality of Reform and Accountability in Today's Public Service.* London: Public Finance Foundation.

Wall A (1989) *Ethics and the Health Services Manager.* London: King's Fund.

The Patient's View, Part I

Angeline Burke, Nigel Ellis and Ben Griffith

In order to gauge the patients' views of the Patient's Charter, one has either to ask a selection of individuals or to turn to surveys. The following two chapters feature both approaches.

The Information Team at the Association of Community Health Councils have written about the surveys and findings that their Association and Community Health Council produces, thus giving a sample of patients' views. Statistics can be produced to strengthen a particular argument and can, therefore, be biased. The authors of Chapter 4 have used their figures in a very even-handed way. Their statistics are, therefore, not simply numbers to take note of but will point readers to the ethical challenges of the Patient's Charter. Each statistic quoted comes with the invitation to see it in terms of what this might mean for patients and their rights, and what it might mean in terms of responsibilities for those who implement those rights.

Chapter 5 gives extracts of three interviews held with people who had recently been patients — or in one case, the mother of young patients. The stories told by these people not only reveal personal views, but also corroborate the statistics of the earlier chapter.

There was no standing ovation when the Health Secretary William Waldegrave announced the Patient's Charter in October 1991. Maybe the analogy drawn in the *Health Service Journal* headline went a little far: 'I have in my hand a piece of paper . . .' (Millar, 1991). However, patients' organisations were none too happy. ACHCEW, the Association of Community Health Councils for England and Wales, said the Charter was a 'big disappointment'. The Patients' Association called it 'rather flabby' and 'gelatinous'. Even the Director of the highly respectable King's

Fund Centre suggested that it was 'something of a middle class charter . . . For a substantial number of people from ethnic minorities or with disabilities or who are homeless, the charter may seem irrelevant' (Stocking, 1991).

On the other hand, the journal *THS Health Summary* concluded that the Government appeared 'anxious for people to have more say in certain aspects of the NHS as a way of improving the service' (*THS Health Summary*, 1991). The RCN was very upbeat about the 'named nurse' concept, the General Secretary describing it as a 'tremendous recognition of the value of nursing'. The National Association of Health Authorities and Trusts (NAHAT) saw the Charter as a first step: 'We need to ensure that the process continues and that targets are extended' (Millar, 1991).

It is still early to take stock, but some preliminary conclusions can be reached about the effectiveness of the Patient's Charter from the patient's perspective, as assessed through surveys conducted by Community Health Councils (CHCs) and their comments on the state of the NHS in their district.

Pre-history

CHCs are well placed to assess the effects of the Patient's Charter. CHCs were set up in 1974 in response to evidence that NHS care was not sufficiently patient-centred. More than 200 CHCs in England and Wales (and similar bodies in Scotland and Northern Ireland) continually press for better standards of health care in NHS contracts, inspect NHS premises and staff at work and help individual patients to exercise their rights and, where necessary, pursue complaints.

CHCs recognised the value of charters of rights long before they became fashionable in Whitehall. ACHCEW

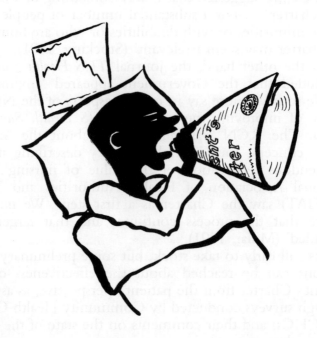

published its own Patients' Charter in 1986 (ACHCEW, 1986). This stated that: All persons have a right to:

1. health services, appropriate to their needs, regardless of financial means or where they live and without delay;
2. be treated with reasonable skill, care and consideration;
3. written information about health services, including hospitals, community and General Practitioner services;
4. register with a General Practitioner with ease and to be able to change without adverse consequences;
5. be informed about all aspects of their condition and proposed care (including the alternatives available), unless they express a wish to the contrary;
6. accept or refuse treatment (including diagnostic procedures), without affecting the standard of alternative care given;
7. a second opinion;

8. the support of a relative or friend at any time;
9. advocacy and interpreting services;
10. choose whether to participate or not in research trials and be free to withdraw at any time without affecting the standard of alternative care given;
11. only be discharged from hospital after adequate arrangements have been made for their continuing care;
12. privacy for all consultations;
13. be treated at all times with respect for their dignity, personal needs and religious and philosophic beliefs;
14. confidentiality of all records relating to their care;
15. have access to their own health care records;
16. make a complaint and have it investigated thoroughly, speedily and impartially and be informed of the result;
17. an independent investigation into all serious medical or other mishaps whilst in NHS care, whether or not a complaint is made, and, where appropriate, adequate redress.

Following the publication of the government's Citizen's Charter, ACHCEW released its 'initial views' on what should be covered by the then imminent Patient's Charter (ACHCEW, 1991). The 21 pages set out, in some detail, reasonable expectations of NHS services in relation to: information for patients; access to services; choice for patients; support; consent; privacy, dignity and respect; rights relating to priority services; complaints and redress; and CHCs. It was perhaps inevitable that the official Patient's Charter turned out to be thinner in content (although glossier in appearance).

- Do governments ever listen to advice given to them?
- Should democratic politicians and neutral civil servants be open to influence by outside organisations?

The Patients' Experience of the Patient's Charter

In theory, *every* citizen is covered by seven established NHS rights which, although they predate the Patient's Charter, are re-emphasised as part of the new initiative. These are given below.

1. To receive health care on the basis of clinical need, regardless of ability to pay

In fact, there is a wealth of documentary evidence that clinical need is not the only determinant of access to appropriate care. Long-standing factors that impinge on access include where patients live and their ethnic group and social class. Recently, the picture has been further complicated by NHS purchasers laying down distinct quality criteria (including waiting time limits inspired by the Patient's Charter) in their contracts with the NHS providers.

CHCs and others have been particularly concerned about the widespread evidence, compiled by organisations such as the BMA and the Association of CHCs, that fund-holding GPs have been able to arrange for their own patients to receive priority treatment in the NHS. The government rejects the relevance of the cases brought to its attention, on the ground that they are not evidence of 'two-tierism'. The official guidance, agreed between the NHS Management Executive and the Joint Consultants Committee, is singularly unhelpful (NHSME, 1991). On the one hand it lays out a number of 'principles' such as, 'timing of the provision of individual patient consultations and/or treatment must be based on clinical need'. On the other hand, 'GP fundholders are explicitly encouraged by the Department's guidance to negotiate variations in the quality criteria that apply in the unit's contracts with its main purchaser. Examples are given of specifications of waiting times, grade of staff treating patients or waiting times in the out-patient clinic'. 'Clinical need' is not, therefore, the only determinant of access to hospital care, even though the 'patient's ability to pay' is not the distorting factor in relation to the NHS internal market.

In other respects, however, patients are increasingly faced with charges for health care, with their associated deterrent effect on those with low-to-moderate income (but not exempted from charges). Prescription and NHS dental charges have increased well above the general rate of inflation. CHCs report that many people have experienced problems gaining access to NHS dentistry as dentists move, where the market allows, towards the more lucrative private sector. Ophthalmic services have been largely privatised. The NHS has largely withdrawn from continuing nursing care for elderly people and others, forcing highly vulnerable individuals into private nursing homes. Lastly, 'private medicine' in the sense of acute surgery has grown dramatically, and some NHS trusts have successfully encouraged the use of their pay beds. If that is not in direct contradiction to the first Patient's Charter right, it is hard to see what could be.

2. To be registered with a GP

Family Health Services Authorities (FHSAs) are legally obliged to find GP services for all patients who come to them having failed to make their own arrangements. However, patients' choice may be extremely limited, particularly in more rural areas. It is also the right of any GP to remove a patient from his or her list without giving a reason. Therefore, those patients who make a complaint about their family doctor (which is their right under the Patient's Charter) run a very real risk of being removed from the GP's list and jeopardising their chances of being registered with a suitable GP practice. It is not just the

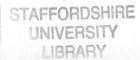

lodging of a complaint that may restrict a patient's right
to be registered with a convenient GP practice; according to the doctors' newspaper *Pulse*, GPs remove patients
from their lists 'when they are too expensive in terms of
the doctor's emotion and time' (*Pulse*, 1994).

The Primary Care Charter, which followed the Patient's
Charter, stated that patients have the right to 'change
doctor easily and quickly'. However, almost three-quarters
of CHCs report that patients experience difficulties, either
frequently or sometimes, when wishing to change their
GP (ACHCEW, 1994a).

**3. To receive emergency medical care at any time, through
your GP or the emergency ambulance service and hospital
Accident & Emergency departments**

The network of emergency services is one of the most
praised aspects of the NHS. However, the Government
has announced changes, made at the behest of GPs, to
reduce the number of visits they make to patients' homes
out of hours. It is much too early to assess the impact of
this. There has also been some 'rationalisation', often
fiercely resisted, of Accident & Emergency departments.
However, new minor casualty units have provided popular
and appropriate care.

**4. To be referred to a consultant, acceptable to you, when
your GP thinks it necessary, and to be referred for a second
opinion if you and your GP agree this is desirable**

The reference to 'second opinions' is one of the most
disappointing aspects of the Patient's Charter, since the
right is conditional on the GP agreeing with the patient.
Also, there is no arrangement for obtaining a second
opinion following a diagnosis made by one's GP — the
only course of action is to find a new GP.

5. To be given a clear explanation of any treatment proposed, including any risks and any alternatives, before you decide whether you will agree to the treatment

Without proper access to a second opinion, what is the patient to do if he or she cannot obtain a clear explanation of proposed treatment? In practice, far more could be done to inform patients about the treatment that is proposed for them and to involve them in choices. Many doctors would go along with the title of the November 1993 article in the *British Medical Journal*: 'Fully informed consent can be needlessly cruel' (Tobias and Souhami, 1993). However, only patients have the right to decide that there are limits to what they wish to know about their treatment and their prospects. There is no harm in recognising the right *not* to know.

6. To have access to your health records, and to know that those working for the NHS are under a legal duty to keep their contents confidential

ACHCEW (1994b) has surveyed CHCs on the Access to Health Records Act 1990, which brought patients' legal rights to see written NHS records broadly in line with their rights under the Data Protection Act 1984 in relation to computerised information. The 1990 Act was undoubtedly a major step forward but a number of limitations have become apparent.

Firstly, the Act restricts access. It does not apply to records made before November 1991. Also, the Department of Health does not regard it as appropriate for patients to see full information about them recorded in the course of the investigation of complaints nor for the patients who have been removed from GPs' lists to be entitled to know why. In other words, some information is not regarded as part of the patient's 'health record'.

Secondly, charges can be levied, which, including photocopying charges, have sometimes been known to be around £50. In one case, a patient was asked to pay £150 to photocopy around ten pages of GP-held health records.

Thirdly, many GPs and dentists appear not to be conversant with patients' rights (where they are not deliberately obstructive): the Medical Defence Union receives around 2500 enquiries each year from GPs and their staff about the disclosure of medical information, records and reports.

Fourthly, the doctors involved play a major role in deciding whether or not the patient should see a record under the Act and, if so, whether the doctor should be present in the room when the record is being inspected. This can be seriously intimidating if, as is often the case, the patient is inspecting the record with a view to complaining about the doctor.

Lastly, there is no independent appeals or complaints machinery so that patients can get a review of a decision that denies or restricts access. In many cases, the decision will be taken (in effect if not in law) by someone who has a vested interest in records being withheld, and that decision is final (except for legal challenge). This is clearly unacceptable.

The main issue in relation to confidentiality is that, in practice, patients' records are seen by many NHS personnel without the knowledge or explicit consent of the patients. In the course of their treatment, a wide range of people who will never exchange the time of day with the patients concerned may need to have access to their records (or would be able to read them over somebody else's shoulder). The records may also be used for teaching, for research or for medical audit, although the information should be 'anonymised' for these purposes. Tight controls are essential if confidentiality is not to be compromised by the easy transfer, copying and storage of information as the NHS becomes more computerised, especially in the context of the internal market, let alone of growing contact with external bodies, such as voluntary and private health-care providers and Social Services departments.

7. To choose whether or not you wish to take part in medical research or medical student training

In practice, this can be a difficult area, and patients are frequently not asked or are placed in a situation in which they feel they have no choice. Patients with a serious but rare disease may be of great interest to medical staff and students; they may feel under great pressure to cooperate, and it is also likely that they will not wish to be obstructive. Patients sometimes find that they repeatedly have to make it known that they do not wish to be inspected by medical students.

• Patients find that even their so-called 'existing' rights are not respected in practice. Does this call for changing the attitudes of NHS staff or giving patients more power?

The Patient's Charter has not only publicised patients' existing rights in the NHS, but also introduced three 'important new rights', effective from April 1992.

1. To be given detailed information on local health services, including quality standards and maximum waiting times

Since the Charter was launched, patients have had access to a wealth of information about local health services, available through the Health Information Service and published as hospital league tables. However, it is open to question whether or not patients can use this information to exercise choice and whether or not they are now more likely to receive accurate and informed answers to their questions.

In practice, there is still substantial room for more, and more useful, information to be made available and for more detail in the quality standards laid down in purchasers' contracts. As more GPs gain fund-holding status, and as the range of services covered by fund-holders' contracts expands, this area will be increasingly difficult to monitor. At present, fund-holders' contracts are supposed to be public documents, but their purchasing plans — which may be more strategic and, therefore, more open to change through realistic consultation — are not. In early 1993, ACHCEW found that 90 per cent of CHCs had never been consulted about fund-holders' purchasing plans and 87 per cent had never even been informed about them. Nearly half of the CHCs that had tried to see contracts struck by fund-holders found this impossible. In practice, many CHCs had been hard pushed to monitor fund-holders: 45 per cent had not sought sight of fund-holders' contracts, and 83 per cent had not attempted to see fund-holders' annual accounts (ACHCEW, 1993a).

2. To be guaranteed admission for treatment by a specific date no later than 2 years from the date when your consultant places you on a waiting list

This may be the area in which the Patient's Charter has had most beneficial effect. Very long waiting times (those in excess of 2 years), between the consultant placing the patient on a list and the patient being treated, have been dramatically reduced. For some operations, including cataract removals and hip and knee replacements, patients should always be treated within 18 months, which has undoubtedly made a vast improvement to the quality of life for those affected. All this is to be welcomed, but qualifications should also be registered.

Firstly, the right ignores the period spent waiting for the initial appointment with the consultant at which time she or he puts the patient on an inpatient waiting list. It is only then that the clock starts ticking, which may be many months after the patient first visited the GP. This has now been recognised by the Department of Health, which aims to set a national target for the length of time people have to wait for their first outpatient appointment, to be laid down from April 1995. There may, however, be a further complication, in that fund-holding GPs may defer referring patients to consultants due to financial constraints; this would be a new, additional and unmonitored type of waiting time.

Secondly, we can ask where the resources come from that have allowed very long waiting times to be tackled. To some extent, they come from the substantial new money granted to the NHS in the early 1990s and from efficiency gains, including possibly lower costs being charged to purchasers as a consequence of the unleashing of the internal market. However, in two respects the gain of the very-long-waiter may be the loss of someone else needing treatment. A year after the introduction of the Charter, CHCs were in no doubt that 'shorter waits were adversely affected in most areas' and that 'cases were reported of priority being given to patients with less clinical need than others' (ACHCEW, 1993a). Also, some purchasers have responded to this new Patient's Charter right by refusing to pay for the treatment of people who could not expect to be treated within 2 years (ACHCEW, 1993b). The Wessex Purchaser Consortium for Plastic & Reconstructive Surgery declared:

> 1.1 All Health Authorities within Wessex Region are required to ensure that by 31 March 1992 no patients will have been waiting for in-patient or day case treatment for more than two years.

1.2 Once targets are achieved purchasers need to have a
clear view of the services they wish to buy from April
1992 onwards. Purchasers who wish to maintain and further
reduce waiting times will need to limit the range of services
purchased.

- Is this a form of NHS rationing that cuts the official
  waiting list by effectively telling groups of people that
  they will wait for ever? Should the NHS strive to
  meet all needs or demands or should some patients be
  told to do without?

**3. To have any complaint about NHS services — whoever
provides them — investigated and to receive a full and
prompt written reply from the Chief Executive or General
Manager**

Moving from the second 'new right' to the third is a step
from the relatively sublime to the completely ridiculous.
It is seriously misleading to say that patients have had the
right since April 1992 to have 'any complaint about NHS
services' investigated. In fact, the formal complaints system
for primary care can only investigate breaches of the
'Terms of Service' — the contract held between practitioners and the local Family Health Services Authority
(FHSA). Important aspects of NHS care, including some
of those covered by the Patient's Charter, are not covered
by doctors' and dentists' Terms of Service. For example,
there is no formal complaints procedure available for
patients that specifically covers a GP refusing them access
to their health records or breaching their right to confidentiality. Even where there is a procedure available to get
a complaint investigated, the reality is that complainants
regularly experience inordinate delays before receiving
proper replies.

The system for dealing with complaints about hospital

and community health services is also subject to unacceptable delays, sometimes stretching from weeks and months to a matter of years when the complaint relates to a clinical matter. Even when a patient's concerns manage to elicit a 'full and prompt written reply', this will be based on an internal investigation carried out by the trust in question and not the report of an independent body. Can this be said to be truly impartial? Even the most serious complaints about alleged clinical errors are considered by two consultants from the same specialty. Lay involvement is not seen as being a necessary component of a satisfactory investigation into a patient's complaint.

Recognising the depth of concern from patients as well as professionals, the government set up a review of the complaints system under Professor Alan Wilson, whose report was published in May 1994 (DoH, 1994). The Wilson Report has recommended that the complex and bureaucratic procedures that have been allowed to evolve in the NHS are replaced by a single unified system for dealing with complaints. This should be speedy and simple to use for the patient, while still providing a full and fair response and/or investigation.

• It can only be hoped that the Department of Health recognises that such a system is necessary. Can a complaints system be fair if it is not independent of both parties? What can 'independence' mean when complaints *about* the NHS are considered *by* the NHS?

It should be clear that patients cannot always be sure that their rights as set out in the Patient's Charter will be respected. The Charter, in itself, has no legal standing, although some of the rights were already established in law. However, having set out patients' rights, the Charter moves on to the 'nine National Charter Standards', which are not claimed to be 'guaranteed' but which 'we are aiming to provide for you'.

1. Respect for privacy, dignity and religious and cultural beliefs

There are obvious difficulties in assessing whether or not a standard such as this is being attained, and how much this is due to the Patient's Charter. Although most CHCs monitor the standard as part of their routine visiting programme, the term 'respect' is both qualitative and subjective, and CHCs often have to rely on anecdotal evidence from patients as the most reliable indicator of whether privacy and dignity are observed during a patient's term of treatment. It is often found that the structural limitations and layout of older hospital buildings are the root cause of many complaints.

CHCs continue to press the NHS for changes in recognition of the UK's ethnic and cultural diversity. This is too often neglected, as shown in a recent CHC survey: although information about privacy and dignity was made available to three-quarters of patients as part of the initial admissions procedures, this was available in languages other than English in less than a third of cases (ACHCEW, 1994a). It is arguable that this means that those perhaps most likely to have special requirements are not being empowered to make these known.

In one respect, the situation with regard to patient choice appears to be deteriorating: financial pressures have led some hospitals away from single sex wards, which many patients, especially women, want because of their medical condition, their cultural background, their personal experience or their reasonable fears of sharing a ward with members of the opposite sex.

Mid Essex CHC conducted a survey at Broomfield Hospital Accident and Emergency Department and found that: 'Nursing staff were more sympathetic and friendly to patients than reception staff, but both groups do not take seriously the patients' need for privacy'. The CHC was 'particularly concerned about a patient's privacy both at the reception desk and when undergoing triage' (Mid Essex CHC, 1993).

Bury CHC's Patient's Charter Monitoring Unit surveyed this standard in February–March 1993. 91 per cent of respondents said they felt they had sufficient privacy during their stay — 'it is difficult to imagine a more positive outcome', commented the Unit. 92 per cent felt that their dignity had been given full consideration — 'very satisfactory', according to the CHC — 65.5 per cent said their religious beliefs had been catered for and 31 per cent did not know. Similarly, with cultural beliefs, 59 per cent felt that they had been catered for and 38 per cent did not know (Bury CHC, 1993a).

2. Arrangements to ensure everyone, including people with special needs, can use services

In the absence of civil rights legislation to provide a suitable environment for disabled people, the important issue of access has been given the status of a standard that the NHS aims to attain, rather than a guaranteed right. This is disappointing both to CHCs and to groups of and for disabled people. CHCs are continually monitoring the accessibility of NHS buildings and finding no shortages of improvements to suggest.

Two members of East Cumbria CHC, themselves with mobility problems, toured the district investigating the accessibility of all the NHS premises. They identified the following problem areas:

Parking — lack of designated parking spaces close to entrances.
Signposting — some could be improved.

Entrances — ramps lacking or steep, no rails, doors difficult, lack of call bell.

Exits — as a safety point, some fire exits were blocked by furniture, mats etc.; some had steps rather than ramps outside.

Floors — often appear shiny, which may be off-putting.

Seats — more seats with arm rests to help elderly infirm people with sitting/standing.

Toilets — toilets either lacking or inadequately equipped for disabled people, e.g. no rails, no lever taps, mirrors etc. at the wrong height.

Rails — rails would improve long corridors.

Call bells — whether at entrances or in, for example, toilets to summon assistance.

However: 'Provider Managers in East Cumbria have reacted positively to the study' (East Cumbria CHC, 1993).

3. Information to relatives and friends

It is again difficult to gauge the impact of the Patient's Charter on the arrangements that exist to inform relatives and friends about the progress of a patient's treatment. However, around 50 per cent of CHCs believed there had been an improvement in this area 1 year after the Charter had been introduced (ACHCEW, 1993a).

Bury CHC's Patient's Charter Monitoring Unit found that 79 per cent of patients at Bury General and Fairfield General Hospitals said that their relatives and friends had been kept informed about their progress while they were in hospital, and 14 per cent did not know. The Unit commented: 'Given that most hospitals have notoriously bad records for communications with patients and patients' relatives, these results must be acknowledged as being excellent' (Bury CHC, 1993a).

4. Waiting time for an ambulance service

The Patient's Charter standard states: 'when you call an emergency ambulance it should arrive within fourteen minutes if you live in an urban area, or nineteen minutes if you live in a rural area'. However, a survey in early 1994 found that one in five CHCs reported that their local ambulance service had been failing to meet the national standards. One in five reported that a reduction in the number of ambulance stations since 1990 had led to longer waits for some local people, and two in five said that ambulance stations in their area had either closed or were at risk of closure (ACHCEW, 1994a).

5. Waiting time for initial assessment in Accident & Emergency departments

'The Charter Standard is that you will be seen immediately and your need for treatment assessed.' In a survey, 17 per cent of CHCs reported that their Accident & Emergency department understood this to mean that patients should be assessed straight away, while another 69 per cent of CHCs reported that the standard was understood to require assessment within 5 minutes. Four-fifths of CHCs reported that the assessment would be made by a specific triage nurse, while another one in ten said an other nurse would assess (ACHCEW, 1994a).

Hillingdon CHC surveyed the A&E Departments at Hillingdon and Mount Vernon Hospitals, interviewing 237 patients at the former and 189 at the latter. Only 72 per cent of patients at Hillingdon Hospital (74.5 per cent at Mount Vernon) were assessed by the triage nurse within five minutes. The CHC concluded that the triage system 'is clearly a success but it needs to be operational for 24 hours' (Hillingdon CHC, 1994).

6. Waiting time in outpatient clinics

The Patient's Charter standard is that patients should be given a specific appointment time and be seen within 30 minutes of that time. This was certainly an area in which progress was needed to stop patients waiting for hours to be seen.

Bury CHC's Patient's Charter Monitoring Unit investigated the Charter standard in August 1992 and April 1993. The 30-minute standard was achieved in relation to 47 per cent of patients, ranging from 32 per cent for Elderly clinics to 60.5 per cent for surgical clinics. 'The Charter Standard achieved in the Out-Patient Department at Bury General Hospital showed a steady improvement and is now very close to 50 per cent, which is the very minimum we should expect.' Overall, 22 per cent of patients had to wait over an hour (Bury CHC, 1993b).

Where delays do occur, patients should not just be left sitting around in outpatient clinics but should be kept informed of the reason for the delay.

• An extension of the Charter standard to this effect would benefit patients and further the 'culture change' so long needed in the NHS. Why does the NHS sometimes appear to place such a low value on *patients'* time?

7. Cancellation of operations

Under the original Patient's Charter, 'The Charter Standard is that your operation should not be cancelled on the day you are due to arrive in hospital . . . If, exceptionally, your operation has to be postponed twice you will be admitted to hospital within one month of the date of the second cancelled operation.' From April 1994, this has been tightened up, so that patients are entitled to be admitted within a month of any operation cancelled on the day the patient is due to arrive in hospital — or, in practice, when the patient has already arrived. Unfortunately, this does not apply when the operation has been cancelled the day before (leave having been arranged from work, child care having been arranged and sleep having been lost), let alone a week before.

8. A named qualified nurse, midwife or health visitor responsible for each patient

It is of course a good thing for patients to know the names of those caring for them, but it is likely that the one named individual will only be at work — let alone free to attend to the patient — for a fraction of the patient's stay in hospital. Good care depends on teamwork as much as on individual responsibility.

East Cumbria CHC surveyed discharge arrangements from local mental health services and reported in passing: 'Nearly all the patients said that they had a named nurse or key worker looking after them. However, it is obviously important, given the major role such a person plays, to ensure that the named nurse is available to the patient as often as possible (2 patients mentioned their key worker was away on holiday or on a course)' (East Cumbria CHC and Community and Mental Health Unit, 1993).

9. Discharge of patients from hospital

To quote the standard in full: 'The Charter Standard is that before you are discharged from hospital a decision should be made about any continuing health or social care needs you may have. Your hospital will agree arrangements for meeting these needs with agencies such as community nursing services and local authority social services departments before you are discharged. You and, with your

agreement, your carers will be consulted and informed at
all stages.'

CHCs have paid close attention to the arrangements
made for patients' discharge, since there is often room for
improvement. The Greater London Association of CHCs
(GLACHC) conducted a survey of discharge arrangements
in late 1993. CHCs reported a wide range of short-
comings, and the report from GLACHC found 'that not
only do we have a "patchwork quilt" rather than the goal
of "seamless care", but that the quilt is full of holes'.
GLACHC organised a discussion day, from which the
'overwhelming message . . . was that there were not sufficient services, providing either health or social care in
the community, to support the numbers of people being
discharged from hospital'. The largest area of complaint
related to people being discharged before they were ready
to go, in that they were still too ill or support services had
not been made available. There were also 'complaints from
users and carers about their lack of involvement in the
planning for discharge . . . relatives felt that patients were
being pushed out of hospital' (Joule, 1994).

East Cumbria CHC's report on discharge arrangements
from Garlands Hospital found some areas of concern; for
example, two-thirds of patients said they had not received
an information handbook, one-third felt their discharge
was not well planned and 'nearly 30 per cent wished to
be involved more'. Generally, however, the results were
encouraging; 82 per cent of patients were satisfied with
the arrangements and planning for their discharge and 51
per cent were very satisfied. 'Perhaps the "ideal" discharge
is summed up by the patient who said: "It was done at
my pace and I was involved and my wishes were taken
into account" ' (East Cumbria CHC, 1993).

It should be noted that the Patient's Charter states only
that patients will be 'consulted and informed at all stages',
not that arrangements for discharge will be subject to

patients' agreement. In one important respect, this formu-
lation marked a step backwards from guidance issued by
the Department of Health in 1989 (DoH, 1989). Indeed,
shortly before the Patient's Charter was launched, the
Government told the House of Commons Social Security
Committee, 'Health Authorities have a responsibility
under the National Health Service Act to provide nursing
care for those who cannot or do not wish to pay for it.
Department of Health guidance is clear that people should
not be discharged into private nursing homes when they
have no wish to pay' (House of Commons Social Security
Committee, 1991). In reality, CHCs have frequently been
contacted by the relatives of patients who felt pressurised
into agreeing to be discharged into nursing homes. In
August 1994, the NHS Executive issued a draft circular,
which, should it come into force, would effectively rescind
the 1989 'clear' guidance and reject the 1991 interpretation of the NHS Act. In this respect at least, the Patient's
Charter has played its part in drawing back the boundaries
of the NHS and taking away from elderly patients and
others their right to nursing care under the NHS.

• Does the ageing of the population mean that there
  will be increasing pressure to cut back the range of
  services available on the NHS to elderly people? Is it
  right to deny care to people who have paid taxes
  and National Insurance contributions throughout their
  lives, in the expectation that they would be helped
  when they needed it?

Local Charter Standards

In addition to setting out national rights and standards,
the Patient's Charter also stated that health authorities
would be increasingly setting and publicising local charter

standards on a range of subjects such as the waiting times in Accident & Emergency departments after the patient's need for treatment has been assessed.

However, in early 1994, 31 per cent of CHCs said that their health authority had not set out local charter standards on Accident & Emergency waiting times. Not all those that were laid down look very impressive: standard maximum waits for non-urgent cases of 2 or 3 hours are common, and one CHC even reported a maximum of 4 hours. One-third of CHCs dealt with complaints about the time that patients were kept waiting in the Accident & Emergency department. One CHC referred to delays of up to 12 hours (ACHCEW, 1994a).

CHCs in London have joined together in 'Casualty Watch', visiting their local Accident & Emergency departments on the same afternoon, specifically to assess the number of patients waiting on trolleys for beds. GLACHC reports that 'A Casualty Watch in March 1994, by four CHCs, found that people at St Bartholomew's and King's College Hospitals faced the longest delays, with 14 people found waiting for a bed for more than six hours — including five people waiting more than 20 hours. It also showed that elderly people faced the longest delays of all. In the April 1994 Casualty Watch 58 people were found, at 13 hospitals, waiting for a bed for more than 3 hours' (GLACHC, 1994).

Public Awareness

The Patient's Charter and the publications under the Citizen's Charter umbrella have been very widely circulated and hyped at the taxpayer's expense. However, an ICM survey published in August 1993 (Shrimsley, 1993) found that just 40 per cent of respondents had heard of the Patient's Charter. However, the National Consumer

Council published a MORI survey in October 1993 that suggested a dramatic improvement: 'The majority, just under two-thirds (64%) of our respondents, say they have heard of the Patient's Charter. But only a quarter (24%) recall seeing one and even fewer — around one in five (19%) — remember reading any of it.' Seventy-nine per cent of respondents from middle-class social groups (ABC1) had heard of the Charter, compared with 53 per cent of C2DE respondents (NCC, 1993).

In April 1994, the Royal College of Nursing published an Audience Selection poll, which again found that two-thirds (69%) had heard of the Patient's Charter. Only 28 per cent of respondents could, however, name any of its rights or standards.

Among those who did know of the Charter, the highest identification rating (13%) was for the half-hour wait in outpatient clinics (standard no. 6), while the named nurse concept was identified by only 1 per cent (standard no. 8). Of respondents who had been treated by a nurse in the previous year, or a member of whose family had been treated by a nurse, just 29 per cent said the concept had been explained to them, and 43 per cent said they knew they had been given a named nurse.

Warrington CHC surveyed local people's views on the Patient's Charter itself. The survey was based on the CHC's 'Health Watch' panel, made up of 420 local people who had expressed their willingness to participate in CHC projects and were likely to be well informed on health matters. The survey found that 77 per cent of respondents were aware of the Patient's Charter, three-quarters of whom claimed to have read the Charter.

Respondents were asked how important was each of the Charter rights. 98 per cent said that right no. 3 (to receive emergency care) was very important, and next came right no. 1 (to receive health care on the basis of clinical need), which 94 per cent rated as very important.

At the other end of the scale was right no. 8 (to be given information), although 57 per cent of respondents thought that very important too. 44 per cent of respondents were not aware that patients' rights are 'guaranteed', and 53 per cent said they would not know whom to talk to if they felt they had been denied their rights. 'The failure to provide adequate information — on treatment, medication, nature of illness and also on anticipated waiting times, is the principal cause of the denial of Charter rights.'

The most popular Charter standard was standard no. 4 (on response times for ambulances), which 95 per cent thought very important. 91 per cent said standard no. 5 (immediate assessment in Accident and Emergency) was very important. The least popular standard was no. 8 (the named nurse, midwife or health visitor), which 54 per cent thought very important. 'Waiting times at clinics, cancellation of operations, unavailability of notes, lack of respect, inadequate services for disabled patients, are quoted as examples of the failure to provide Charter standards' (Warrington CHC, 1993).

- Which of the Patient's Charter rights and standards are most important and which are less important?
- If patients have different priorities from health-care professionals, what does that mean? If it comes to a choice, who should decide?

Revision of the Charter

In April 1994, the Secretary of State for Health announced that a revised Patient's Charter would be issued that autumn. The Patient's Charter Unit at the NHS Executive consulted the Association of CHCs and said that new standards and targets were being worked up in five areas:

1. a national target on waiting times for inpatient treatment for coronary artery bypass grafting;
2. a national standard for waiting times for a first outpatient appointment;
3. a national standard on hospital catering services;
4. a national standard on timed appointments for community nurse visits;
5. a national standard on information about admission to a mixed sex ward.

In its response, ACHCEW recognised that the Patient's Charter had acted as a tool for improving health-care services. However, the Association suggested a dozen areas to be addressed by a new Charter:

1. Everyone should have the right to be registered with a dentist under the NHS.
2. The right to a second opinion should be strengthened.
3. Patients should have firmer rights to inspect information kept on them by the NHS.
4. Confidentiality issues need to be addressed in the context of developments in information technology, clinical audit, the internal market and community care.
5. More information should be published, for example about hospitals' readmission and postoperative infection rates and about fund-holders delaying referrals for financial reasons.
6. Patients' ability to use the published information to choose between providers needs to be enhanced.
7. Patients should normally be able to choose a doctor of their own gender.
8. Disabled people should have the right to use services independently, rather than relying on help from others.

9. Advocacy and interpreting services should be available by right.
10. Maximum waiting times should be set for treatment in Accident & Emergency departments.
11. All patients needing continuing nursing care should be entitled to receive that care under the NHS.
12. Patients should have the right to the support of a relative or friend at any time.

In addition, ACHCEW endorsed the need for a national right to have any complaint about the NHS investigated and a full and prompt reply received. There was an urgent need to bring NHS practice in line with the undertaking in the Patient's Charter if the latter was not to be drawn into disrepute.

Conclusion

The early 1990s was a period of dramatic change in the NHS. The operation of the internal market and the associated establishment of NHS trusts and GP fund-holding, a major input of new resources and the introduction of the Patient's Charter all created new interest in the quality of and access to NHS care. It is not possible to separate out the practical effects of these three aspects of government policy, nor have the consequences all enhanced patients' rights. The NHS has increasingly withdrawn from 'non-priority' treatments and from continuing nursing care.

* Does this mean that the patient's right to receive NHS services — the most important health care right of all — has been significantly undermined? Is it fair to blame the Patient's Charter?

There is, however, little doubt that the Charter has laid down minimum standards and encouraged NHS providers to rise above those standards. The push from the Department of Health at the centre has been supported by the NHS purchasers (health authorities, commissioning agencies and fund-holders) as the purse-holders, along with CHCs and other patient representatives. In theory, the internal market may, on its own, have forced standards up, although it has created an additional pressure to force costs down, not always with happy consequences. As the argument over fund-holding has made clear, improvements generated by the internal market inevitably raise issues of equity and may conflict with the principle of providing services according to need.

- Does equity matter? If a few NHS patients get better services, is that a good or a bad thing?
- Can the national Patient's Charter be a mechanism for improving standards across the board, without causing the inequities that have caused resentment and raised serious ethical issues?

For all its defects, the Patient's Charter did not deserve the widespread contempt with which it was greeted. There is a lot to be said against it — but we would be worse off without.

References

ACHCEW (Association of Community Health Councils for England and Wales) (1986) *Patients' Charter — Guidelines for Good Practice*. London: ACHCEW.

ACHCEW (Association of Community Health Councils for England and Wales) (1991) *From 'Citizen's Charter' to 'Patient's Charter'*. London: ACHCEW.

ACHCEW (Association of Community Health Councils for England and Wales) (1993a) *Annual Report 1992/3*. London: ACHCEW.

ACHCEW (Association of Community Health Councils for England and Wales) (1993b) *Rationing Health Care: Should Community Health Councils Help?* London: ACHCEW.

ACHCEW (Association of Community Health Councils for England and Wales) (1994a) *Annual Report 1993/4.* London: ACHCEW.

ACHCEW (Association of Community Health Councils for England and Wales) (1994b) *Access to Health Records Act 1990: The Concerns of Community Health Councils.* London: ACHCEW.

Bury CHC (1993a) *Charter Standards Report No 3.* Bury: Bury CHC.

Bury CHC (1993b) *Charter Standards Report No 4.* Bury: Bury CHC.

DoH (Department of Health) (1989) *Discharge of Patients from Hospital.* London: HMSO.

DoH (Department of Health) (1991) *The Patient's Charter.* London: HMSO.

DoH (Department of Health) (1994) *Being Heard — The Report of a Review Committee on NHS Complaints Procedures* (Wilson Report). London: HMSO.

East Cumbria CHC (1993) *Getting Round the Health Service.* Carlisle: East Cumbria CHC.

East Cumbria CHC and Community and Mental Health Unit (1993) *A Quality Initiative to Examine Discharge Arrangements from the Mental Health Services.* Carlisle: East Cumbria CHC.

GLACHC (Greater London Association of Community Health Councils) (1994) *Casualty Watch.* Briefing no. 20. London: GLACHC.

Hillingdon CHC (1994) *A Survey of the Accident and Emergency Departments of the Hillingdon Hospital and Mount Vernon Hospital.* London: Hillingdon CHC.

House of Commons Social Security Committee (1991) *The Private Financing of Residential and Nursing Home Fees*, HC 421, Session 1990/91. London: HMSO.

Joule N (1994) *London Hospitals — Discharging their Responsibility?* London: GLACHC.

Mid Essex CHC (1993) *Results of Survey — Accident & Emer-*

gency Department — Broomfield Hospital. Chelmsford: Mid Essex CHC.

Millar B (1991) 'I have in my hand a piece of paper . . .'. Health Service Journal, 101(5277), p. 12.

NCC (National Consumer Council) (1993) Consumer Concerns 1993. London: NCC.

NHSME (National Health Service Management Executive) (1991) Joint Guidance (NHSME/JCC) to Hospital Consultants on GP Fundholding, EL(91)84. London: NHSME.

Pulse Editorial (1994) The real reason GPs strike off patients. Pulse, 54(29), p. 27.

Shrimsley R (1993) Nearly one in three has never heard of the Citizen's Charter. Daily Telegraph, 26 August, News.

Stocking B (1991) Patient's Charter. British Medical Journal, 303 (6811) pp. 1148–9.

THS Health Summary Editorial (1991) The spirit or the letter? THS Health Summary VIII(XI) p. 1.

Tobias J S and Souhami R L (1993) Fully informed consent can be needlessly cruel. British Medical Journal, 307(6913), pp. 1199–1201.

Warrington CHC (1993) Health Watch Project — Report of the Survey on the Patient's Charter. Warrington: Warrington CHC.

The Patient's View, Part II

Verena Tschudin

The story and the two interviews that follow speak for themselves. The three individuals concerned are introduced briefly at the beginning of their sections, but a word about their participation is also called for.

The selection of these particular people was very deliberate. Thelma had told me her story just after it happened, and I asked her to retell it for this chapter as it is an example of what happens when one person consciously claims one of the rights in the Patient's Charter. Sandra and James have been known to me for many years, and I asked them to be interviewed because both of them had had contact with hospitals since the Charter had been published. Their stories and approaches to the Charter are very different. They do, however, confirm some of the findings in Chapter 4, that about two-thirds of people have heard of the Charter, although only a quarter have seen it and fewer still have any idea what might be in it. This begs the questions of whether the effort of implementing the Charter has been worth it, whether it is effective, who or what might help to make it effective and whether this would actually help?

The Patient's Charter is mostly concerned with rights — and, therefore, with responsibilities — and these stories show yet another aspect of these elements. They are individual stories, but they are also universal stories, which may evoke responses from readers and their clients and students.

My particular thanks go to Thelma, Sandra and James (whose names and identities have been disguised) for giving their time and views.

Thelma

Thelma is 48 years old, a university lecturer, keen on sport and in very good health. She is well acquainted with the Patient's Charter and, indeed, with most of the charters produced in the last years. She had quite a collection of them to show me. She told me the following story.

I had this small growth at the side of my face, which came and went, and every time that I thought it would disappear, up it came again. I guessed that it was nothing very serious, but, when I went to my GP for a routine appointment, I mentioned it to him, and before I knew where I was, he was writing a referral letter to a cancer dermatologist at my local hospital. He told me that he thought it was a rodent ulcer, that it was malignant but not invasive, but that I must definitely have it looked at. He gave me the letter to take to the hospital, which I could do easily.

I went, therefore, to the hospital outpatients department and eventually located a window that had 'New Patients' written over it. At the other side of the window was a computer, and two women were working in the background. Eventually, one of them turned round and came towards me. She was leaning over the computer to speak to me. She took the letter from me, opened it and began to read it. At this stage, I began to be alarmed and said that surely this letter was from one doctor to another and that she was breaking confidentiality by reading it. She told me that she needed to read it to have details of my address. I told her that I could have given her my address verbally as I was capable of speaking. She was mumbling something about this being normal procedure.

I was not going to take this lightly. I knew the Patient's Charter and knew that one of the three new rights was 'to have any complaints about NHS services — whoever provides them — investigated and to receive a full and prompt written reply from the Chief Executive or General Manager'. So I wrote to the Chief Executive, having made sure that I knew his name. I quoted to him the first of the Charter standards, which provides for 'respect for privacy, dignity and religious and cultural beliefs'. I wrote that I did not think that my 'respect for privacy' was maintained that day and that presumably, if a procedure is being followed, everybody else subject to this procedure is not having their dignity respected.

About 3 weeks later I got a letter from the acting manager of the outpatients department. She said that she was sorry that I had been offended and then said she regretted that sometimes the process seems more important than the patient. You can say that again! Anyway, she went on to say that, apart from personal details, the appointments clerk also needs to know whether the GP thinks that the appointment is urgent and whether it should be for a specific clinic run by the consultant. She assured me that all staff in the NHS work under a rule of patient confidentiality but that there must be communication between members of staff so that appropriate services can be provided. The letter ended with a line to say that she would be discussing my concerns with the staff involved so that no further distress should be caused; if I had any further concerns I could phone her. I thought a letter would be better, because I just did not think that an appointments clerk should be in any position to decide what steps to take. If the GP knew what to do he would have done so, but he referred me to a consultant — not to a clerk.

I received another letter, telling me in detail what the procedure is, but I cannot understand this: in one paragraph, the letter states that a letter is flagged up to the consultant if the GP writes that an appointment is urgent, and in the next paragraph it says that the consultant decides what is required. I am still left with the impression that the appointments clerk is the one who makes the decisions on what kind of treatment the patient should get in the first instance. The acting manager expresses her sorrow again that I felt that, on becoming part of the system, confidentiality goes out of the window. I had not actually used that expression, but, in the circumstances, I thought it was ironic to use these words, when all this started with a transaction through a window.

I just sent a note to acknowledge the letter; I didn't think that I would get anywhere if I took this further. What more could I have done, or, for that matter, what should I have expected? But I must admit, I have always had my suspicions about hospitals and confidentiality. This is only a little incident, and in the end, I am sure that I am not actually harmed. But the system worries me, and the loss of dignity and respect, too. It's fine to have charters, but the more I come anywhere near them, the more I think that they are a complete waste of money. We should have these rights anyway — we should not have to fight for them or be told in a high-handed way that we are lucky to be given them.

- Was Thelma right to complain?
- Thelma complained about confidentiality — what about the lack of respect shown to her?
- Should she have left the matter where and when she did?
- Has anything changed because of her action?

Sandra

Sandra is 35 years old and the mother of two little boys. She was a paediatric ward sister until about 6 years ago. The older of her boys recently had to be hospitalised. Sandra also told me that she had heard of the Patient's Charter but had never seen it. The following is an edited version of that interview.

Author: Have you heard of the Patient's Charter?
Sandra: I have heard of it, but don't know its content.
A: What do you think should be in it?
S: I feel that it should be to do with the individual rights of the patients, as opposed to what the doctors think is best for them.

It should be about what the patients think is best for themselves and about the rights they have to know about their treatments.

A: Are you thinking that it is specifically related to treatment?

S: Yes, treatment and information; diagnosis and treatment, expectations, choice of treatment and care and where this is going to be.

A: This is pretty close — that's how it ought to be!

S: What sort of rights should somebody have?

A: You mentioned some — do you think there are others?

S: Well, I think that each patient has a right to respect and dignity. Perhaps they are not the things that ought to be written down, but perhaps they are. These are the things that I should take for granted if I were the nurse giving the care or the patient receiving the care. And the right to privacy. That gets down to basics, doesn't it?

A: Do you think you had different care recently when you took Godfrey [the older son] to hospital, which might be attributed to the Charter?

S: I also took Clement [the younger son] to hospital about 3 years ago, and I feel that the care I received has changed between then and now. I now do also voluntary work at the hospital, on the children's ward. So I am seeing care again from a different perspective, and I think that 3 years ago, as the mother, I did not get the support I needed. With Godfrey it was better; he was receiving more individual attention, but now I have been working as a volunteer twice a week at the hospital, I feel that it has not improved at all and that there is a great need for improvement.

A: What about your GP? Have you noticed any difference in care there?

S: Yes, my GP practice has changed in the last 2 years. I have got to know them quite well over the last few years, and they have told me how they are trying to change it, which may have influenced how I have received this. They have more rules and regulations. They are trying to achieve certain targets. There are notices around saying that you should not wait for more than 20 minutes, and if you do, you should let them know, which has all obviously to do with the Patient's Charter and the rights of the

patients. I have received very good care from the GP. When I had
a breast lump and had to go to X— Hospital, it was all done very
quickly. I had something else recently that I thought needed
attention, and within 3 weeks I had an appointment at Y—
Hospital. I thought that was impressive. I feel that that would not
have happened 2 years ago.

A: So, overall would you say that you have seen improvements in
the GP practice?

S: Yes, but not so much in hospital. In the last 3 years, there has
been a slight improvement, but I don't think it has been enough.
It was noticeable last time that all the children had their parents
with them, and if they didn't, the children were bored or lonely.
We felt very strongly that Godfrey had to have somebody with him
all the time in case he needed anything. We were not sure that
a nurse would always be there to deal with his needs. We were
also encouraged to be there. We had a nice room, and there
was a proper Z-bed there and a bathroom for both of us to use,
so it was easier. There were no parents sleeping on chairs, as
occasionally happened when I was still working.

A: There is a sense now that people should complain more since
the introduction of the Patient's Charter. How quickly would you
feel willing or able to complain?

S: If I felt there had been a shortfall in the care or the advice I
had been given, or that it was wrong or could have been avoided,
I would complain straight away. Who I would complain to is
probably the next question. I don't know who you are supposed
to complain to, but I would ask.

A: What would you complain about?

S: I can't think of anything personal, and even with two children
in hospital, I have never complained. We were kept in Accident &
Emergency for a very long time when I took Clement into hospital
3 years ago, and that irritated me, but I didn't think it was worthy
of a complaint. If I felt that drugs were given wrongly, I would
complain about that.

As a volunteer, I have twice come across parents who have
been in hospital for 5 days with their sick children and nobody
had told them that there was a canteen downstairs in the basement

where they could have a meal. That I think is wrong, and I felt inspired to write to the sister on the ward and suggested that I write a leaflet for the parents, which can be handed out. That is an example of what I would do. The parents have a right to be told that sort of information.

A: Do you think that it is because you are a nurse that doctors and nurses relate to you differently anyway?

S: They do; they tell me more. I went with my mother-in-law to see a consultant physician about her sciatica, and he told her what he was going to do, and she didn't understand it. I asked the questions for her because I knew that he was not being clear, and if I had gone as a patient, I don't think he would have given me such a wiffly-waffly answer, because I would not have accepted it. If you are articulate and intelligent, you can state your case better. I have heard so many parents sit in silence and then say to me afterwards, 'What was he talking about?' Perhaps they are not bright enough, but also doctors have such an aura.

A: Information-giving and receiving always concerns me: it should be given unconditionally, irrespective of how intelligent you are or how good you are at asking questions. Those who can't ask questions need the information even more.

[I then handed Sandra a copy of the Patient's Charter, and as she browsed through it, she noticed Charter standard no. 7 about cancellation of operations. She picked this up and said:]

S: Cancellation of operations — now it would be interesting to see whether that is working . . . if I need a particular operation, I would be interested to know what the anaesthetic death rates were in that hospital before I went to have my operation there. Godfrey was circumcised when he was 5 months old, and I had heard that the anaesthetic risk at Z— Hospital was far less, statistically, than that at the local hospital. I have this real fear of anaesthesia, and it was then 1 in 80 000 at Z— Hospital and 1 in 20 000 at the local hospital, so the GP got us into Z— Hospital. This was easy because I had worked there and he could write that I was a former nurse and would like the child treated there. As those statistics were made available for me, I used them. Statistics can help if they are used in relation to everything else.

A: But then a lot of people would not have that information.

S: No.

A: Do you think that such information should be more widely available?

S: I think so.

A: Where would you make it available?

S: I suppose it has to be at the GP's, where the patient is first seen.

A: Or should it be the GP who says, 'I think he would be better off in that hospital rather than in this one'?

S: I think GPs have a lot to do at the moment, anyway, that is not patient care. But they should have that information, yes. My GP works incredibly hard, I know. She takes her medical literature to bed as bedside reading so that she can keep up to date.

A: Thank you very much, Sandra, for sharing your views with me.

- Does it matter that Sandra did not know what was in the Patient's Charter?
- Should Sandra, as a volunteer working in a hospital, know what is in the Charter in order to help her clients?
- Is it right that Sandra, as an ex-nurse, can use her influence with her GP to have information of statistics and get to the hospital she trusts most? Is the principle of justice devalued or strengthened by this?

James

James is a 73-year-old retired inspector of a bus company. He has only been home a few days after a second hip replacement operation. I had asked him if he were willing to be interviewed, because I knew he had strong opinions mixed with a good dose of humour. When I told him it was about the Patient's Charter, he said, 'You mean that

thing Major put forward?' When I switched the tape
recorder on, James started straight away with:

James: The thing is, as an ordinary sort of consumer, or customer,
it is incumbent upon us as patients to be as useful and
cooperative and helpful as we possibly can, bearing in mind that
we are not the only people with problems. But I am digressing
slightly . . . When I came out of the operating theatre and regaining
consciousness . . . the woman in the bed across said, 'Well, I'm
glad you are a man. The last time we had a woman and all she
did was moan, moan, moan'. So I did my best to be cheerful.
There is nothing like a hospital for understanding and
comprehending human nature, both from its humorous and its
pathetic side.
Author: So, to the Patient's Charter, have you heard of it?
J: I have heard of it.
A: But you don't know what it is?
J: Well, it's a bit of political propaganda, as I see it, although
whatever the government do, either as individual ministers or
collectively, there must be a politically ideological basis. But the
vast majority of people have reacted by saying, 'Well this is just
another gimmick and there is not much in it for us'.
A: What do you actually think it is?
J: Well, it is a good idea. It is worth pursuing. It is probably
prohibitively expensive but would be justified if it could be made
to work without political infighting and that sort of thing. I am
digressing slightly. It would be a d . . . good thing if the NHS
were taken away completely from government and run by a
national trust, but that is only a personal opinion.
A: Well, but a good one. What do you imagine then is actually in
the Patient's Charter?
J: History has reflected all too certainly that those who have,
manage, and those who have not, simply do not. And over the
past 200 years or so, since trade unionism, politically informed
bills and what have you, there has been some restoration of
balance. But as always, there are far more poor people in the
world than there are rich, and, as the Lord put it, the poor will

always be with us. But mankind and society in general, and politicians in particular, have got to redress this imbalance between those who have and those who have not. It is being achieved slowly, particularly in Britain and the more enlightened nations of Europe, Sweden, perhaps, and Holland, but they are having the same problems, aren't they? — the cost.

But it has got to be run in the future, and, as I said, it would be far better done if it were a national trust of highly competent and properly trained administrators of the old, pre-war type. There used to be widows, of the war . . . and they used to form trusts around hospitals, Princesses and the like, when I was a little boy, and these old dears used to come round on Sunday afternoons and shake your hand, and even then you always felt that you were part of the thing. Mind you, childhood memories are pretty strong. But nevertheless, from an ideal point of view you can see that this — is empathy the word? — between nurses, doctors, patients and so on, is essential from the patients' point of view. And I pull no punches, dear, it is sadly lacking, from my experience, in the X— Hospital.

The purpose of it . . . Well, that is the idea. As Beveridge put it, in his 1944 Act, medical aid should be available to all, irrespective of position and income, which is a noble idea. And I mean, when I got married and my children were born, which is 40 years ago, things worked splendidly. The district nurse came to the home. There was none of this controversy raging now about giving birth in hospital; it wasn't done. There was a system of NHS midwives, day and night. You rang the doctor, or you rang the nurse, and the nurse came once a day, twice a day. The doctor came. The whole thing ran smoothly. Now it involves God knows what, forms and appointments . . . It is the inevitable consequence of science, of course, the inevitable problem of cost. So, ideally, the function is that the people should know and be convinced, and this conviction should be based on their own experience, that if they need treatment, from a broken ankle to a headache, from the doctor, or suitable service, they should have treatment irrespective of their social and economic circumstances. That is

the ideal. So, I have no quarrel with the idea. How it is applied
of course is another matter. Is that a sufficient answer?
A: Would you say that you have noticed a difference in your care
in hospital or from your GP?
J: Well, you use the word difference. The word difference implies
a comparison. Now, prior to my first hip in 1991, my last affliction
was haemorrhoids in 1977, which was done very well in the old
Y— Hospital, and there was a continuity or empathy, because of
the nature of this . . . it required a daily dressing. The sister or
whoever who would be doing the dressing . . . we had a chat,
and you would ask how you were progressing and how the wound
was, and she would say, yes the wound is good, you have a
good healing flesh, so you came away all the more confident and
secure and comfortable. But in the X— Hospital, every sister
and there seemed to be far more than needed, and two or three
nurses and auxiliaries, all doing their various jobs, all went
around . . . it was only the chat between the patients that kept the
place going. I tell you this in all honesty, and include it if you
can.

One of the more regrettable developments in recent years in
pursuit of social justice and all the rest of it, is this ghastly
concept of demarcation. You get this impression that all these
sisters, nurses and auxiliaries are allocated by union agreement,
a division of jobs. They start at A and finish at Z, and that is that.
And I give you an example, also off the record. I don't know if I
told you about this grand plan of intensive home nursing.
A: Yes, you did.
J: And I may also have told you that 2 days after I had my
operation, one of the girls who had made all these wonderful
plans came and said, 'I'm sorry, Mr D, the whole thing has been
scrapped. So instead of going home, you will be kept in hospital,
and we will no longer be responsible for you, but the hospital will
ensure that you are fit when you leave'. I wasn't. It was decided by
someone that I would come out last Monday. Someone also
decided the time. Someone also booked an ambulance. You
require 48 hours notice to get an ambulance. Anyway, at 12
o'clock, without telling me or my sister, or my brother, or anyone

who was on duty at that time, in rolled a man with a trolley and
said, 'Mr D, you are on your way home'. I had no pants on, I was
still in my pyjamas, I knew nothing about it. My sister knew nothing
about it; she was out for about 2 hours, she couldn't be found
and my brother couldn't be contacted because he was out at
work. No-one could get into this flat. So there was a great panic.
Well, one of the sisters said, 'You will have to stay another 2 days,
that's another £1000 for the X— Hospital, but we'll see if we can
fit you in later in the afternoon'. They did, and I came home only
to find that the gas company had taken all the pavements up,
and the ambulance had to stop in the road, with a great pile of
rubbish, and they had to carry me over that and up the steps.
But that sort of thing should not happen.

A: Some people have seen the Patient's Charter as rights they
now have, and if these are not fulfilled, they complain. They see
it as a tool for complaining.

J: Well, this of course is another one of the unfortunate
characteristics of human nature. Being, thank God, reasonably
blessed with a balanced mind and attitude, I am inclined to regard
whatever is done in the world by people as individuals or
collectively as for the good of human nature as well. But not
everyone thinks that way. There are people who see an opportunity
to be critical, and not just critical but pejoratively critical. They stir
up any hornets' nest that happens to pass by, to their advantage,
and I think that is tragic. That is another unfortunate aspect of the
political scene.

A: What sort of things would you complain about?

J: Well, slovenliness by the staff, whether they are professionals
or not. I can recall in 1977, when I was in the old Y— Hospital,
they were developing an antiseptic. It is on the market now, but
in those days, it was still being developed. It is a white, clear
liquid, odourless, but it is very efficient. A ward orderly, I suppose
you would call her, would come around to wipe the bedside
locker whenever it was necessary. She came in every day, she
put this flannel in the water with this solution in and followed the
contours of every piece of equipment that was on the table. Now
that is slovenliness.

A: But if you actually had a real complaint, would you take up pen and paper?

J: Well, if it got bad enough, yes. That, of course, is one of the faults of not only hospitals. They say that the trouble with things that go wrong, trade, commerce and so on, is that people do not complain, so the bad habits continue. Although I would, in fact, probably be a bit hesitant, I think that these matters should be brought to the immediate attention of the supervisor. Yes, I would. But if you do, you immediately become a bit of an outcast. You don't want to become a martyr, and you don't want to become a source of controversy.

A: I have a copy of this famous Charter. Would you like it?

J: I'll let you have it back later.

A: You can keep it.

J: The cynic always . . . the first law is: present an image! And the second law is: make that image as attractive as possible to those whom you are about to address. And you get nice presentation, attractive colours, splendid lay-out, good prose, but nothing about what you are actually trying to do! But what they actually do . . . there are lots of long-winded words like 'liaison with', 'cooperation with', 'extensive negotiation with' . . .

A: This is a good summary!

J: And, of course, they have taken their cue from the mail order system. You know as well as I do: £100 000 can be yours! . . . It is not all bad. It is like an edifice that has beautiful architectural contours, but the bits in between are not there.

A: Thank you very much, James, for your honest views and reactions.

- Is James typical of most elderly people in mistrusting the Patient's Charter?
- When pressed, James seemed very reluctant to complain if necessary; is this right, given his attitude, or should everyone be encouraged to complain?
- Should James have made a complaint about his discharge from hospital?

Endpiece

The Patient's Charter is not *the* answer to the present difficulties in health care. Some people would argue that it has only made these difficulties worse; indeed, this may be implied from certain comments in the present text. It is a cliché to say that history will prove it right or wrong, but it is probably the truth.

At one level, the Charter has started a groundswell of discussion about rights, and these have to be considered. When people are given rights, they want and need to use them; but are these in the Charter really rights — and the appropriate rights?

Rights can be divisive and split the population even more into those who have or claim the rights and those who are to provide the rights or see that they are provided. Yet, what our society needs is not more division and individualism but cohesion, working together and a sense of community that is caring in its essence. It is questionable whether the Patient's Charter will bring this about.

At another level, the Charter is no more than a piece of paper that is irrelevant for most people. If so few people have heard about it or know what it consists of, what was all the fuss about? Nothing has changed — or at least, nothing has changed for the better, say the cynics. But are they right?

Many professional health-care workers up and down the country have tried to make the Charter relevant for themselves and their clients and patients. Discussions have been started and new ways of considering themselves and their clients have been sought. Whether this is enough is questionable, but it is a start.

Ethics will always be about what 'is', what 'should be' and the tension between them. Ethical debates are raging at the boundaries of the known or the possible. The

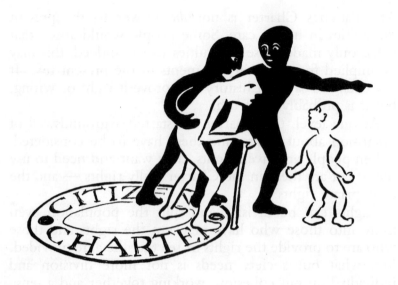

boundaries will always extend, and ethics will, therefore, always be necessary. The present climate in health care will change and is changing. The direction it takes will depend not only on a few policy makers, but also on each one of us. This often seems impossible in practice, when one seemingly gets nowhere (as Thelma's story implies). Too often, people feel that their efforts are useless and wasted, and apathy is, in the end, easier. Ethics calls for people with wide views and wide commitments, which can be applied in 'narrow' ways, i.e. in individual cases and situations. The lived experiences of individuals need to come together in the 'story' of the community and the nation, for the good of the one and the many. It is hoped that the 'story' of health care will be enhanced with the contribution made by the people in this book.

Index